# THORACIC OUTLET SYNDROME FOR PATIENTS AND NON-PHYSICIANS

# THORACIC OUTLET SYNDROME FOR PATIENTS AND NON-PHYSICIANS

Explained in layman's terms for patients and practitioners

Dr. Richard J Sanders
and
Dr. Stephen J Annest

ISBN: 1508570590
ISBN 13: 9781508570592

# Table of Contents

# Acknowledgment

Our thanks to Alexis Petracek and Jo Sanders for their assistance and critique in preparing this book.

# About the authors

Dr. Richard Sanders is a vascular surgeon who has treated many patients with thoracic outlet syndrome over the past several years. He is clinical professor of surgery at the University of Colorado Health Science Center. In 1991, he authored a book entitled "Thoracic Outlet Syndrome: A common sequela of neck injuries". He has also authored more than 30 papers on the subject of TOS which have appeared in medical journals and more than 30 book chapters on TOS which have appeared in surgical text books. He lives with his wife in Denver Colorado.

Dr. Stephen Annest is a vascular surgeon who has treated many patients with thoracic outlet syndrome for several years. Dr. Annest graduated from University of Washington School of Medicine , interned at Virginia Mason Hospital, completed a residency in General Surgery at Albany Medical college and then graduated from a vascular surgical fellowship at Baylor University Medical Center in Dallas, Texas.

He became interested in thoracic outlet problems and their treatment while working as attending vascular surgeon at the Guthrie Clinic in Pennsylvania. In 1995, he moved to Denver where he worked for 3 years with David Roos, a pioneer in TOS and the surgeon who devised the transaxillary approach to brachial plexus decompression.

In 2009, Dr. Sanders and Dr. Annest joined forces in order to collaborate on patients who suffer from the group of disorders known as Thoracic Outlet Syndrome. They have been treating patients together since then with the goal of educating physicians and patients about the diagnosis and treatment options for that group of problems and of improving the care and outcomes of those patients.

# Author's Preface

This book is written in response to patients' requests for more information about TOS in layman's terms. In the following pages, medical terminology has been simplified and explained. Included are descriptions of specific disorders involving the nerves, arteries, and veins of the upper extremities. Many of the disorders are due to injuries to the neck and arms while some are attributable to congenital cervical ribs or abnormal first ribs.

The book will be of help not only to patients and their families but also to practitioners in allied medical fields including nurse practitioners, physician assistants, physical and occupational therapists, personal trainers, and athletic trainers, especially those in the fields of baseball, volleyball, and weight training. Attorneys and legal assistants who deal with neck and upper extremity trauma may also find this helpful.

# Introduction

Thoracic Outlet Syndrome, abbreviated TOS, is a medical term that includes a group of separate conditions which lie in the same area of the body, but have little else in common. "Thoracic" is the Latin word for chest. The "Outlet" of the chest is the area in the neck, behind the collarbone, where the blood vessels from the heart leave the chest going to the neck and arms. This area is called the thoracic outlet area. There are many different types of syndromes in medicine and other fields. A medical syndrome is a group of symptoms or physcial complaints that occur together. For the thoracic outlet syndrome, the syndrome part is pain, numbness, tingling, and weakness in the upper extremity due to pressure, behind the collarbone, against the nerves and blood vessels (artery and vein) going to the arm. Because there are three separate types of structures involved, nerves, arteries, and veins, there are 3 different types of TOS.

In addition, the same nerves, arteries and veins involved above the collarbone, continue below the collarbone to pass under the pectoralis minor muscle. The pectoralis minor muscle can exert pressure against essentially the same nerves, arteries, and veins seen above the collar bone, but since the pressure is now coming from below the collar bone under the pectoralis minor muscle (PMM), these conditions are labeled pectoralis minor syndrome (PMS).

This publication will deal with each of the 3 types of TOS and 3 types of PMS.

# Three types of TOS and PMS

There are three types of thoracic outlet syndrome depending on whether the pressure against the nerves, vein, or artery, lies above the collarbone or below the collarbone. The terms used to describe each type are:

**Neurogenic**--referring to nerves
**Venous**--referring to veins
**Arterial**--referring to arteries

Using these terms, there are 3 types of thoracic outlet syndrome, from pressure above the collarbone, and 3 types of pectoralis minor syndrome, from pressure below the collarbone. These are:

1. **NTOS**—Neurogenic type of TOS; **NPMS**—neurogenic type of PMS
2. **VTOS**—Venous type of TOS; **VPMS**—venous type of PMS
3. **ATOS**--Arterial type of TOS; **APMS**—arterial type of PMS

These terms and abbreviations will be used throughout this monograph. Refer back to them when necessary.

## INCIDENCE

Of all TOS cases, over 90% are neurogenic TOS (NTOS) and/or neurogenic PMS (NPMS). Much less common, about 3-5%, are subclavian and axillary vein obstruction giving rise to venous TOS (VTOS) or venous PMS (VPMS). Least common is arterial injury causing arterial TOS (ATOS) or arterial PMS (APMS), occurring in less than 1% of all TOS patients.

# Part I

# Brachial Plexus Compression: NTOS and NPMS

## INTRODUCTION

Injuries can occur to the nerves and blood vessels (called the neurovascular bundle) of the arm and shoulder above or below the collarbone. Above the collarbone injuries occur in the thoracic outlet area while below the collarbone they are under the pectoralis minor muscle. Injuries in these areas produce thoracic outlet syndrome (TOS) or pectoralis minor syndrome (PMS). It is common for both the thoracic outlet and pectoralis minor areas to be involved simultaneously in the same patient, something referred to as a double crush syndrome[1] (**Upton 1973**).

## CLASSIFICATION

Currently, all types of TOS involving nerves are classified as either neurogenic TOS or neurogenic PMS, depending on whether the nerve compression (squeezing or applying pressure) is above or below the collarbone. In the past, some authors have subdivided NTOS into 3 types: true, disputed, and traumatic (following an injury). True NTOS was defined as NTOS with objective findings (findings one can see, not relying on what the patient feels), by x-ray studies, nerve studies (EMG), and physical findings of muscle atrophy (shrinking muscle). Disputed NTOS was defined as patients with the same symptoms but no objective findings. However, this classification of NTOS has been abandoned by most physician treating NTOS patients because this subdivision of NTOS is no longer useful and the terms "true" and "disputed" has been discarded.[2] (**Illig 2013**) Another reason for eliminating the terms is that it implies that the patient's condition is not real, which is not true because it almost always is real.

## ANATOMY

The anatomical contents of the neurovascular bundle (nerves and blood vessels to the arm) remains essentially the same as the bundle passes from above the collar bone, in the thoracic outlet area, to below the collarbone into the subpectoral area (the area below the pectoralis minor muscle). In this passage, the nerves and blood vessels make few changes other than giving off a few small branches. However, names of the blood vessels change from subclavian above the collarbone to axillary below the collarbone while the group of nerves to the arm are collectively called the brachial plexus, which remains the same name above and below the collarbone. After passing below the pectoralis minor muscle, the brachial plexus separates into individual nerves. Muscles surrounding the neurovascular bundle are all different as the bundle descends from the scalene triangle, through the costoclavicular space (the space between the collarbone and first rib) and under the pectoralis minor muscle. (**Figure 1A**).

The scalene triangle consists of 2 sides formed by the anterior and middle scalene muscles with the first rib forming its base (**Figure 1B**). Inside the triangle are the roots and trunks of the brachial plexus and the subclavian artery. The subclavian vein lies just in front of the anterior scalene muscle, but is outside the triangle.

The neurovascular bundle then passes below the collarbone and above the first rib into the costoclavicular space. This space may be important in VTOS, but its role in NTOS is probably minimal. (**Figure 1C**). Passage under the pectoralis minor muscle, in the subpectoral space, is the next space of importance, more important then the costoclavicular space.(**Figure 2**)

## FIGURE 1: ANATOMY OF THORACIC OUTLET AND PECTORALIS MINOR AREAS

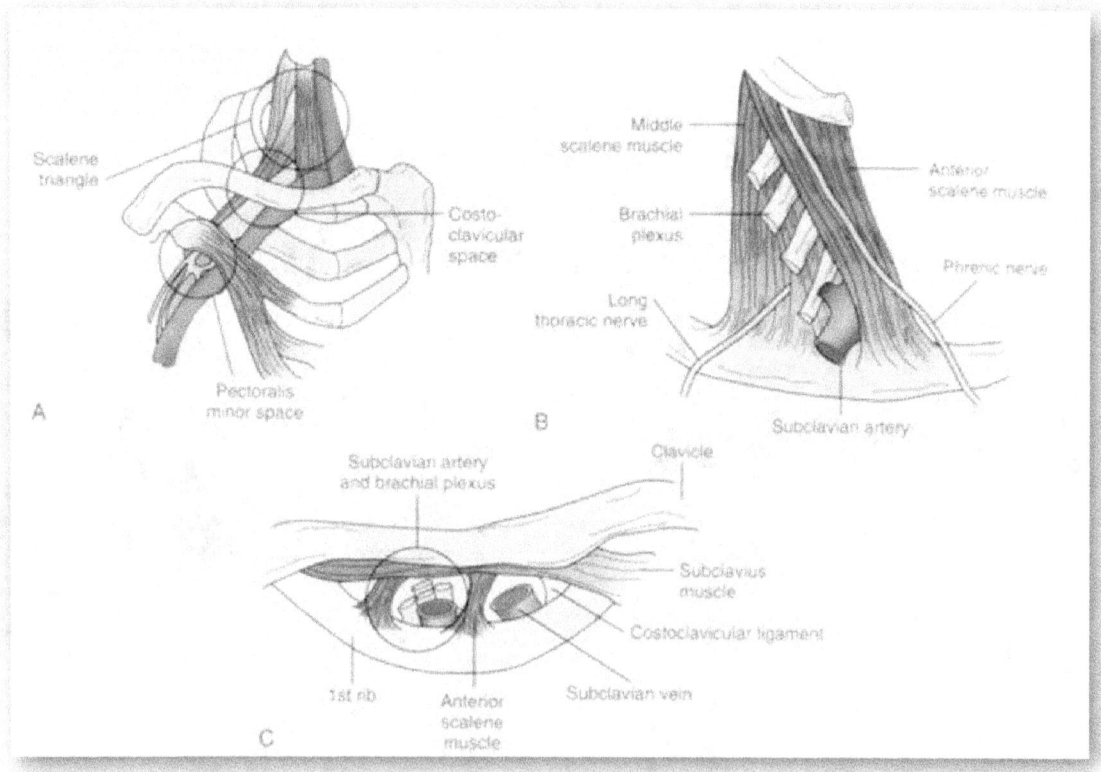

**Figure 1: A. The three spaces in TOS and PMS: B. Scalene triangle C. Costoclavicular space (space between collarbone and first rib).**

## FIGURE 2: PECTORALIS MINOR SPACE

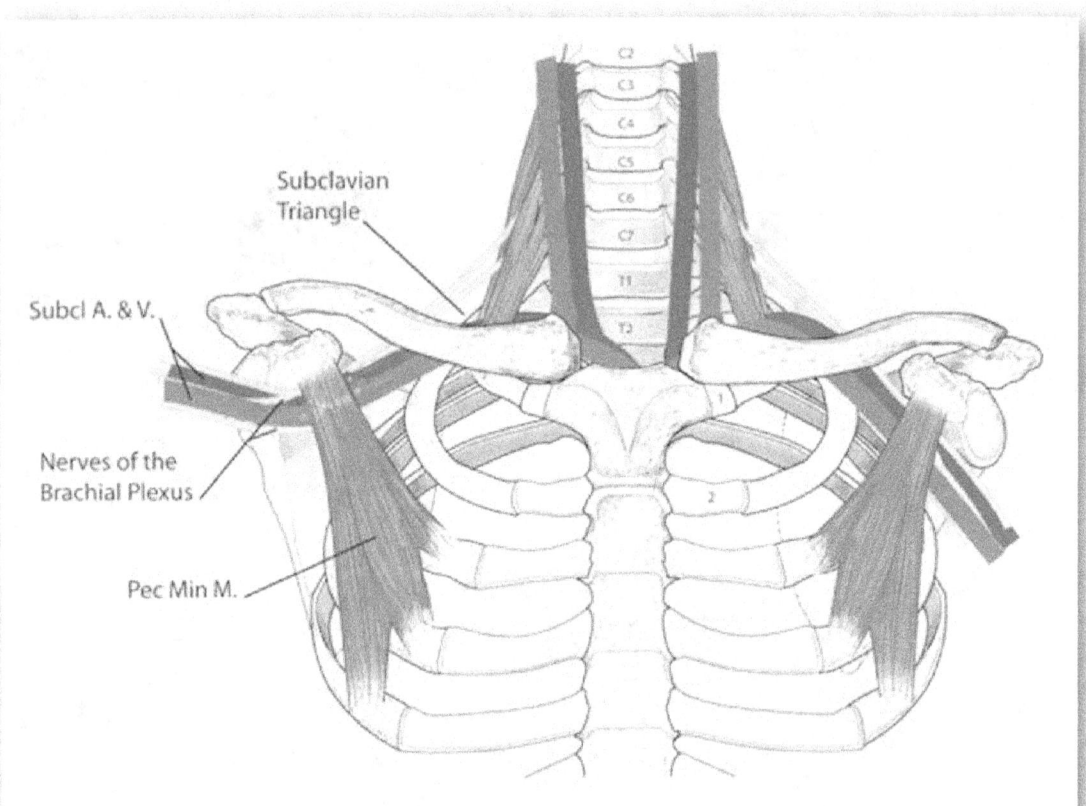

Figure 2: The pectoralis minor space lies under the pectoralis minor muscle
(Pec Min M). The coracoid process (not labeled) is the point of attachment of the pectoralis minor muscle and lies just below the collarbone on the drawing. The coracoid process is an extension of the shoulder blade (the scapula).

Subcl A & V = subclavian artery and vein.

## ETIOLOGY (CAUSE)

The several causes of NTOS and NPMS include acute trauma (injuries) to the head and neck, falls down stairs, on ice or on slippery floors, repetitive stress activities such as typing on keyboards, and congenital cervical ribs or anomalous first ribs.

NTOS is caused by hyperextension neck injuries (the head is forced backwords); NPMS is caused by activities that pull the shoulder blade back (the scapula), thereby stretching the pectoralis minor muscle. (**Table 1**). Both types of stretch-injuries can occur from the same accident.

The shoulder strap of seat belts can injure the pectoralis minor mucle lying below it. Supporting evidence that the shoulder strap can traumatize (injure by an accident) the pectoralis minor muscle, is the observation that drivers of cars with seat belts over their left shoulder more often develop left NPMS while passengers in the same accident more often develop right NPMS.

Tumbling down stairs, or falling on slippery floors or icy sidewalks, frequently causes shoulder injuries along with hyperextension neck injuries. The immediate pain from the shoulder injury often predominates so that the injured person does not become aware of the symptoms from the neck injury until a few weeks, or even months, later. This is why a detailed history of all injuries should be obtained from patients complaining of hand numbness or tingling.

Repetitive stress injuries (RSI) occur from a variety of activities. Sitting and typing on keyboards or keypads are common. Workers on assembly lines, doing the same motions for several hours a day, and grocery store stockers and cashiers are other examples of occupations subject to RSI.

**Competitive sports** is another area where repetitive activities with the upper extremities can lead to nerve symptoms. This is the most common area for teenagers. In this category, the most frequent patients seen are swimmers, volleyball players, baseball throwers, weight lifters, and people who exercise doing large numbers of pushups. All of these are examples of putting considerable strain on the scapula (shoulder blade), which in turn, stretches the pectoralis minor muscle.

**Predisposing factors**: Predisposing factors are anatomical conditions present since birth. Cervical ribs and abnormal (anomalous) first ribs (**Figures 3 & 4**) are primarily predisposing factors which make a person more likely to develop symptoms should neck injury occur. However, some patients with these abnormal ribs become symptomatic without previous injury, in which case the abnormal rib, (or the predisposing factor) is the etiology.

Congenital rib abnormalities, cervical and abnormal first ribs, are often incorrectly regarded as the most common cause of TOS. Cervical ribs are uncommon, occurring in 0.7% (about one in one hundred forty people) of the population. Cervical ribs are twice as common in women as men.[3] (**Haven 1939**) The large majority of cervical ribs are asymptomatic and most patients with cervical ribs will live out their lives without being aware of their congenital extra rib.

An elongated C7 transverse process of the cervical spine (in the neck) is another congenital variation that is often accompanied by a ligament or band. These congenital bands run from the tip of the C7 transverse process (**Figure 3**), through the belly of the middle scalene muscle, to attach to the first rib. Other congenital bands are also seen in the middle scalene muscle and these too usually act as predisposing factors.

Patients with these predisposing factors usually remain free of symptoms until neck injury occurs.

## TABLE 1

## ETIOLOGY OR CAUSE OF NEUROGENIC TOS AND PMS

1.  Neck trauma causing hyperextension injuries (over-stretching backwards)
    A.  Auto Accidents-- rear-end collisions causing whiplash injuries
    B.  Falls down stairs, on ice, on slippery floors
    C.  Repetitive Stress Injuries (RSI)—working on keyboards, assembly lines, weight lifting
    D.  Cervical and anomalous first ribs—put pressure against the lower trunk of the brachial plexus (nerves to the arm) causing symptoms in the 4th and 5th fingers
2.  Competitive Sports—Swimming, volleyball, baseball, football

**Predisposing factors**

1.  Cervical ribs
2.  Anomalous first ribs
3.  Elongated C7 transverse process
4.  Fractures of the collarbone or first rib with callus formation

## FIGURE 3: CERVICAL AND ANOMALOUS FIRST RIB

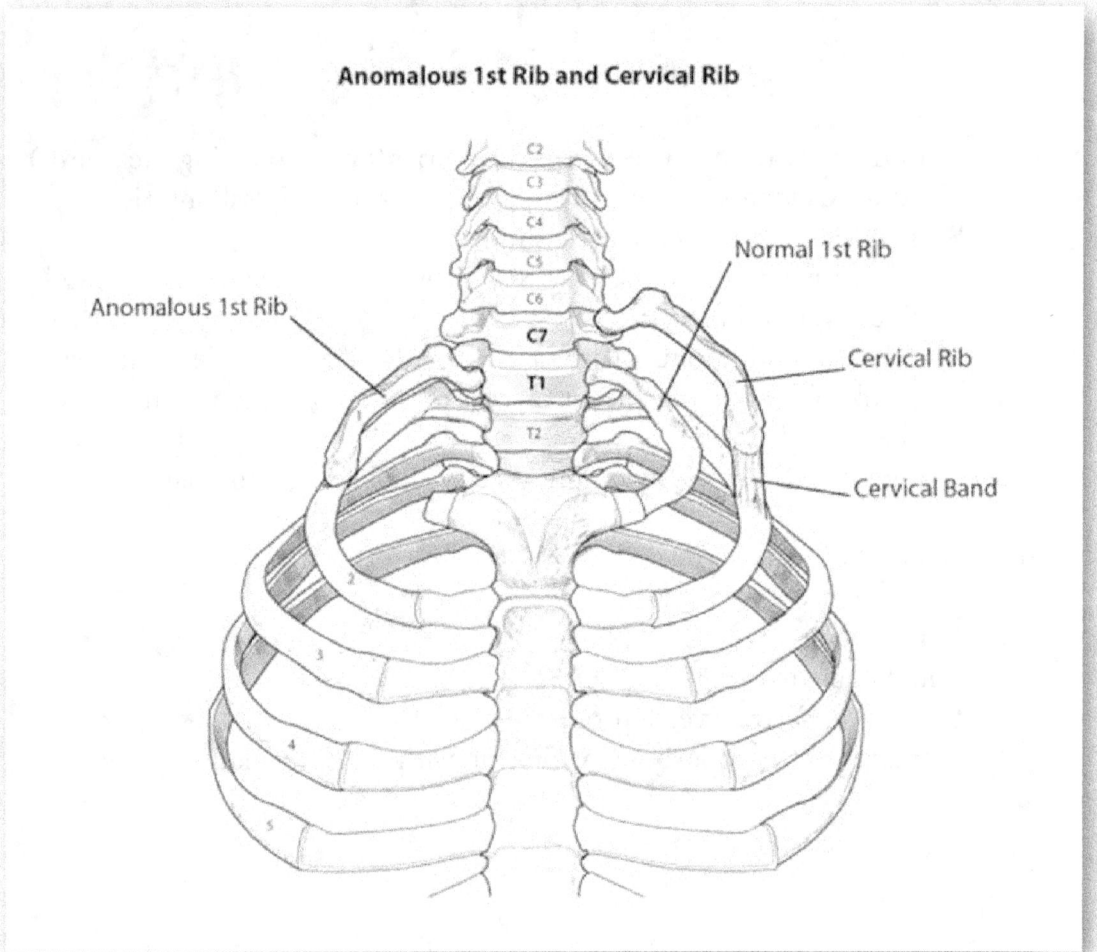

Figure 3: Rib cage showing anomalous first rib the on right arising from the spine at the transverse process of T1; on the left, a cervical rib arises from the transverse process of C7 Also note that from the tip of the cervical rib a congenital cervical band is seen connecting the tip of the cervical rib with the second rib.

FIGURE 4A.   COMPLETE CERVICAL RIB

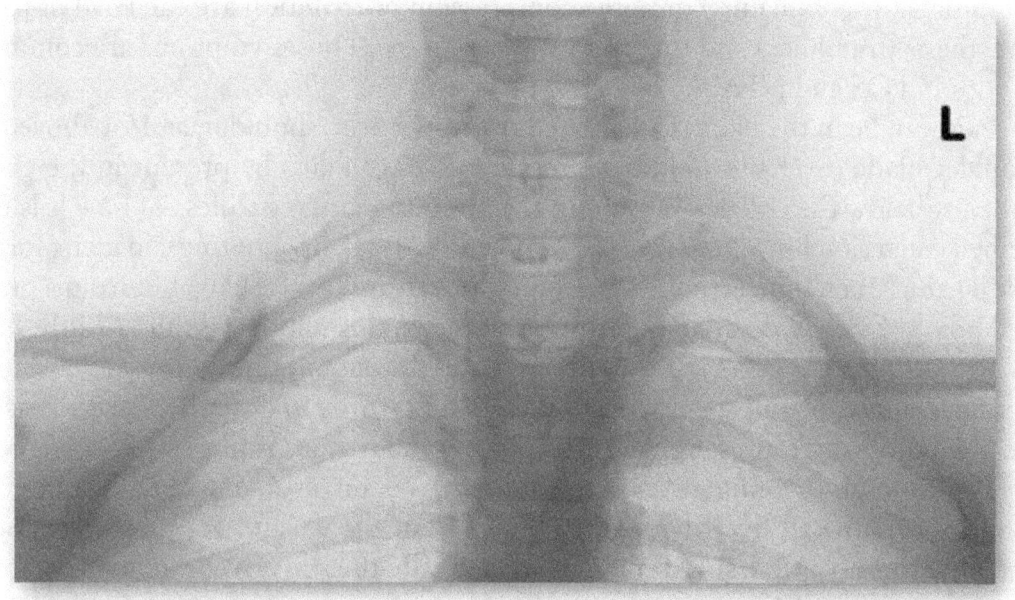

FIGURE 4B.   ANOMALOUS FIRST RIB

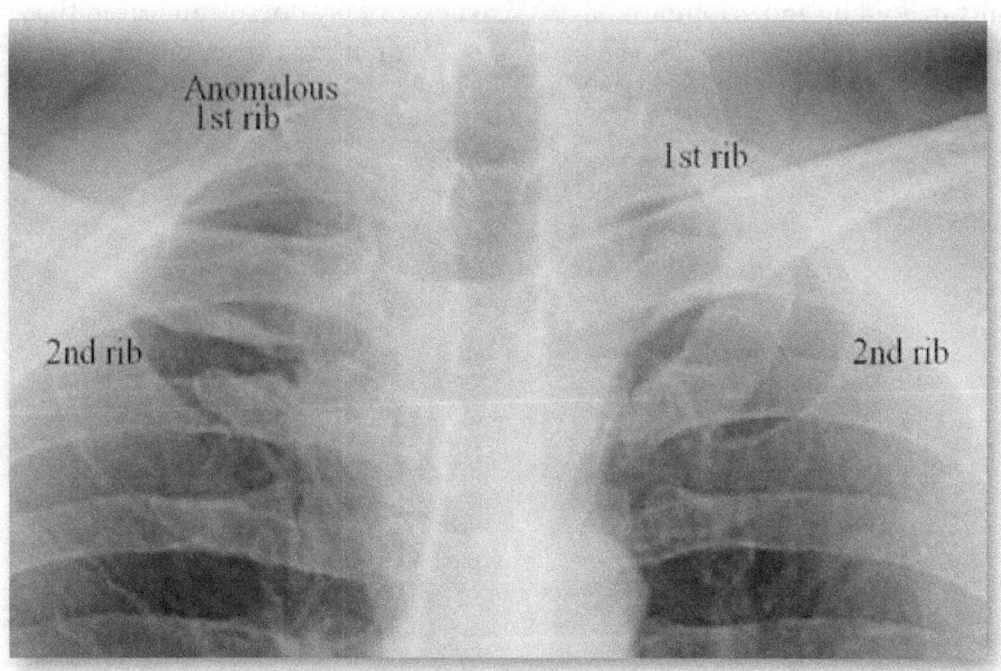

Figure 4:  A.  X-ray of a complete cervical rib with true joint to first rib on the right;
B. X-ray of an anomalous first rib on the right.

## SYMPTOMS

Symptoms (or complaints) of nerve compression or irritation are the triad of pain, paresthesia (numbness and tingling), and weakness. These symptoms are common to both NTOS and NPMS.

**Pain** can be in the hand, forearm, elbow, upper arm, shoulder, and/or above the shoulder blade (over the trapezius muscle). Pain can also be present in the chest wall, just below the collarbone, and in the armpit. Pain, regardless of how it is described (such as aching, general "discomfort", burning, or shooting), in all its forms is still pain. Much time is spent describing the "nature" of the pain, but from a practical point of view, a detailed description of the pain is seldom useful. **(Table 2)**

**Paresthesia** is a good word to describe numbness and tingling as well as other "funny feelings" people experience but can't find words to describe. Paresthesia in the hand most often presents by involving a combination of fingers. Involvement of just the 4th and 5th fingers is quite common as is involvement of all five fingers. In many patients all five fingers are involved but the 4th and 5th are worse. Less often the thumb and first two fingers are the only ones involved. Less often, too, numbness and tingling can involve the forearm and upper arm along with the hand.

**Weakness** is evident by complaints of dropping things from the hand or difficulty in holding and gripping things. Weakness usually doesn't appear until symptoms of pain and paresthesia have been present for at least several months.

## TABLE 2.

## SYMPTOMS OF NEUROGENIC TOS AND PMS

1. Pain (or soreness)
   1. Neck
   2. Trapezius muscle (above the shoulder blade)
   3. Supraclavicular area (just above the collarbone)
   4. Chest just below collarbone over pectoralis minor tendon
   5. Ampit (axilla)
   6. Shoulder
   7. Upper arm
   8. Elbow
   9. Forearm
   10. Hand
2. Paresthesia (numbness and tingling)
   1. All five fingers
   3. 4th and 5th fingers
   4. 1st to 3rd fingers
3. Weakness
   1. Hands
   2. Arms

# Distinguishing NTOS from NPMS

There are differences in symptoms between NTOS and NPMS. In NTOS occipital headaches (in the back of the head) and neck pain are often prominent complaints, while in NPMS, occipital headaches and neck pain are absent or minimal. In contrast, NPMS patients have pain and/or tenderness in the anterior chest wall below the collarbone and in the armpit. If these symptoms are absent, NPMS probably is not present.

NTOS and NPMS coexist when significant symptoms of occipital headache and pain in the neck, plus pain in the chest and armpit, are all present.

## PHYSICAL EXAMINATION

Physical examination for brachial plexus compression is extensive, involving over 20 maneuvers. It includes tenderness over several muscles and a positive Tinel's sign (eliciting pain or tingling down the arm when finger tapping over a specific nerve). In addition, there are four provocative maneuvers (movements that bring on symptoms that are absent at rest) which are specific for brachial plexus compression. While no single positive physical finding is diagnostic of brachial plexus compression, finding several positive responses on physical examination is highly suggestive.

The four provocative maneuvers, which are given that name because they provoke or bring on the patient's symptoms, are also listed at the bottom of **Table 3 and Figures 5,6,&7**. Of these maneuvers, the upper limb tension test (ULTT) is the single, most helpful test.[4] **(Elvey 1986)**. If the ULTT is negative, the diagnosis of brachial plexus compression is highly unlikely in either the thoracic outlet or pectoralis minor areas. False negatives are rare.

## TABLE 3

## PHYSICAL EXAMINATION FOR NEUROGENIC TOS AND PMS

A. Areas of Tenderness (pain elicited by exerting pressure over and area)
  1. Anterior Scalene muscle located in front of neck, next to wind pipe
  2. Biceps and rotator cuff tendons at the shoulder
  3. Trapezius and Rhomboid muscles located over the back above the shoulder blade
  4. Pectoralis minor muscle located just below the collar bone
  5. Axilla (armpit)
  6. Elbow over the ulnar nerve located at the inner epicondyle (prominent bone)
  7. Forearm mucles (radial on top, pronator teres on inside)
B. Tinel's sign is eliciting pain or tingling down the arm by tapping over a muscle or ligament where a specific nerve runs. Tinel's sign is sought in the following areas:
  1. Anterior scalene muscle (next to the wind pipe)
  2. Carpal tunnel (at the wrist)
  3. Medial epicondyle (at the inner elbow)
  4. Pronator tunnel (inner side of forearm)
  5. Radial Tunnel (on top of the forearm)
C. Provocative Maneuvers (movements that bring on symptoms of pain or paresthesia)
  1. Upper Limb Tension Test (ULTT) (**Figure5**)
  2. Neck Rotation (**Figure 6A**)
  3. Head Tilt (**Figure 6B**)
  4. Elevated Arm Stress Test (EAST) (**Figure7**)

## FIGURE 5: UPPER LIMB TENSION TEST (ULTT)

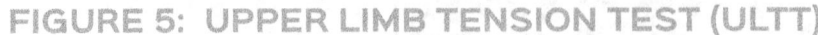

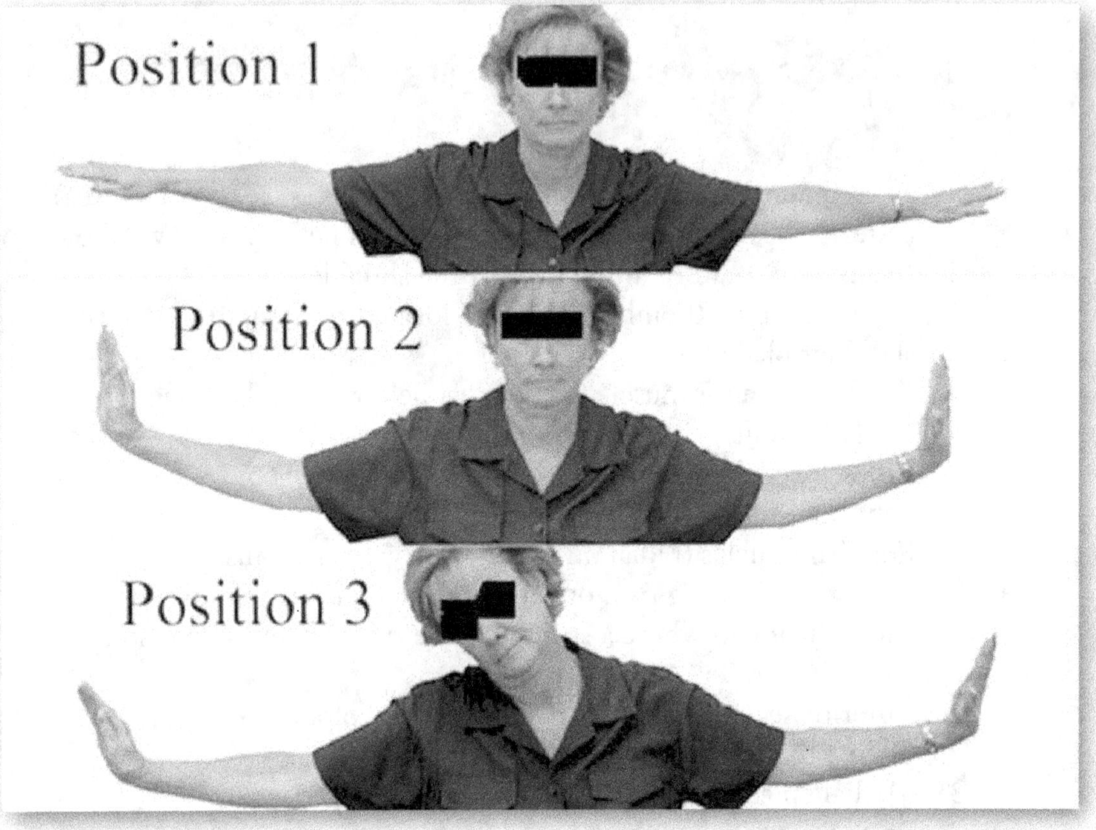

Figure 5: Upper Limb Tension Test (ULTT).

1. First position—Arms at 90⁰ from the body, elbows extended straight out
2. Second position—Wrists dorsi-flexed, towards the ceiling
3. Third position—Head tilted. (this elicits symptoms on the side opposite the tilt)

FIG 6. A. NECK ROTATION

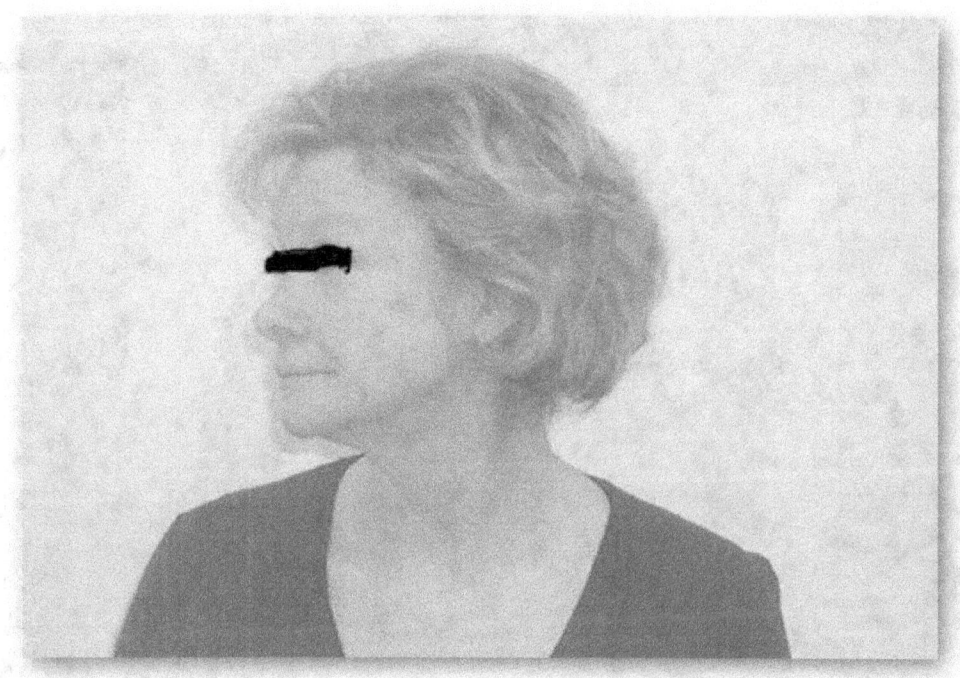

FIGURE 6B. HEAD TILT

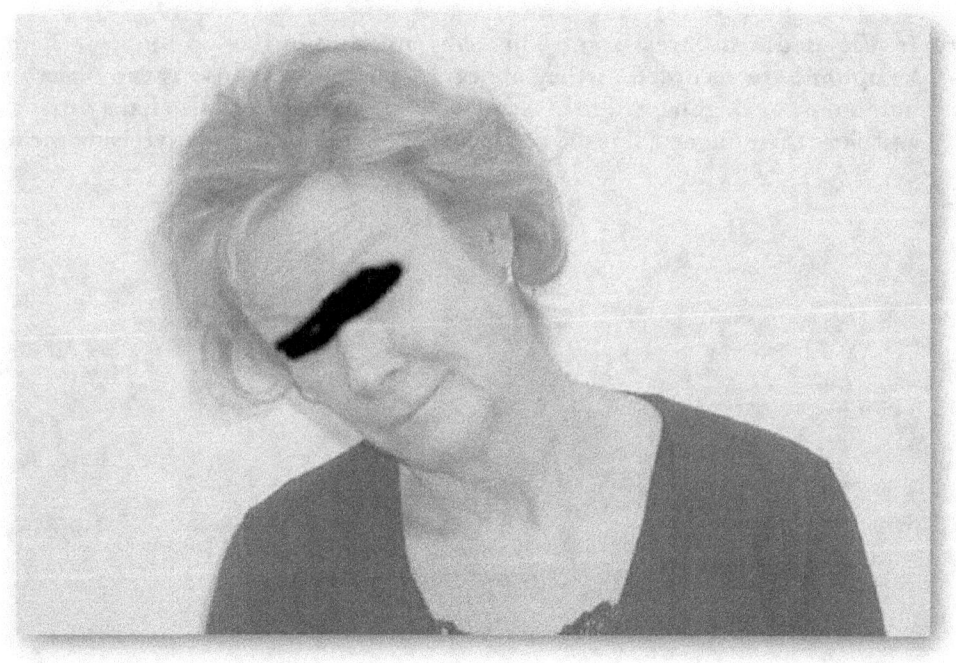

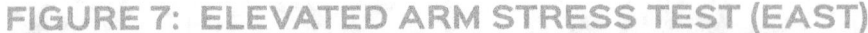

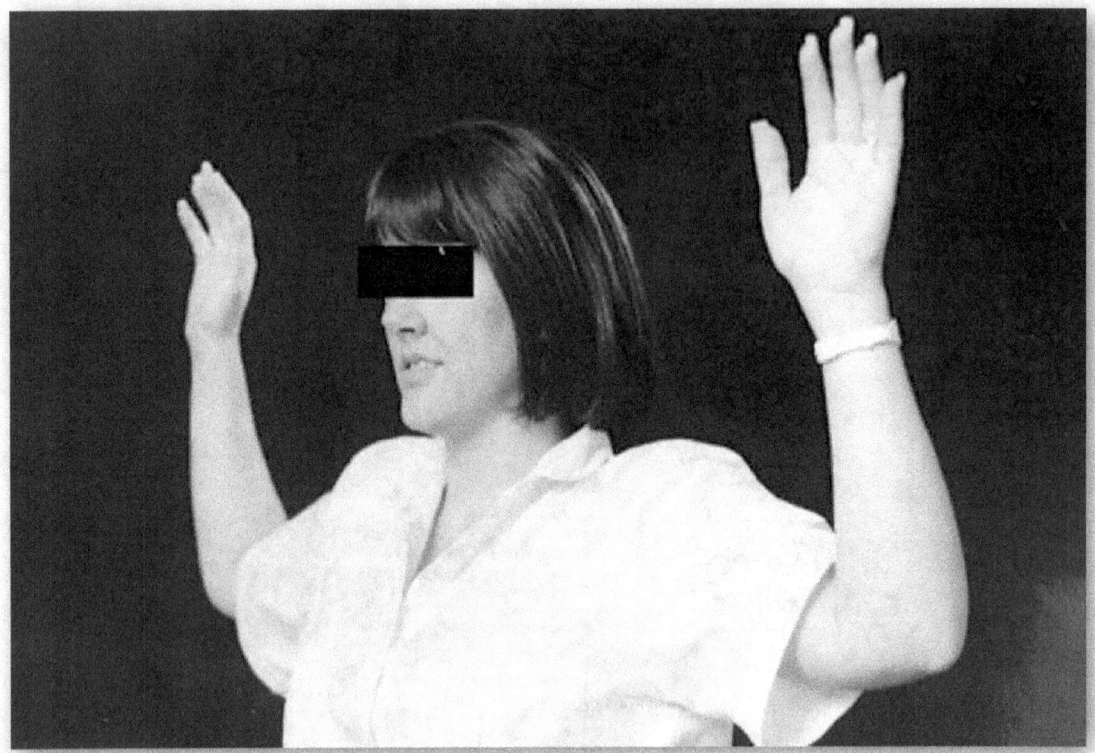

Figure 7: Elevated Arm Stress test. The arms are held in this position for 3 minutes. Symptoms are recorded as they appear. A positive response is the onset of pain, numbness, or tingling within 60 seconds. Some examiners also have patients open and close their fingers. But the test is just as effective without exercising the fingers.

**Adson maneuver:** In 1927, Adson introduced his famous maneuver that is still taught over 85 years later[5] (**Adson 1927**). The Adson test is performed by feeling the radial pulse (at the wrist) of the symptomatic side while the patient's head rotates to the same side, and the patient takes a deep breath. A positive response is a decrease or absence of the radial pulse and the onset of the patient's neurologic symptoms of pain, numbness, or tingling, in that extremity. Over time, many teachers have forgotten about the neurologic symptoms and simply emphasize the decreased pulse. Unfortunately, this test is no longer recommended because several investigators have demonstrated that too many people without symptoms cut off their pulse with this maneuver while too many symptomatic patients fail to do so. [6,7,8,9,10] (**Gergoudis, Warren, Colon, Plewa, Nord 1980-2008**) This happens because the test is relying on a **vascular** sign to diagnose a **neurologic** condition.

The symptoms of pain, numbness, tingling, or weakness are common to nerve compression in several areas of the upper extremity. These areas include the wrist, forearm, elbow, pectoralis minor space, as well as the thoracic outlet area or even the cervical spine. For this reason, physical examination should routinely survey each of these areas to detect tender spots and positive Tinel's signs. Positive responses at the wrist, forearm, and elbow may be due to nerve compression in their respective areas, or they may be due to compression in more proximal areas (closer to the center of the body), such as the pectoralis minor space or thoracic outlet. Another possibility is that there may be compression in more than one area of the upper extremity. This has been described as Double Crush Syndrome[1] (**Upton 1973**). Common double crush situations are the combination of NTOS with Carpal Tunnel Syndrome or ulnar nerve compression at the elbow (Cuboid Tunnel Syndrome). Another double crush combination is NTOS and NPMS. The significance of a double crush syndrome is that it is sometimes possible to relieve symptoms by treating just one of the areas and the other area may become asymptomatic or elicit minimal symptoms.

## DIAGNOSTIC TESTS

### Muscle blocks

Muscle blocks, performed by injecting local anesthetics into a muscle, are very helpful in confirming a diagnosis of brachial plexus compression. The block is performed with the patient either lying down or sitting up. It can be performed with or without ultrasound guidance. Some practitioners have employed brachial plexus blocks for the same purpose as the muscle blocks. We disagree with such usage. A brachial plexus block is a nerve block which renders the arm numb and totally weak. If effective, it will eliminate all sensation and movement from asymptomatic people as well as patients with brachial plexus compression. Because we are looking for a disease process located in muscles, blocking nerves won't tell us if the pain is caused by scarred, entrapping muscles.

Muscle blocks are only performed over tender muscles. Most patients seen for symptoms of brachial plexus compression demonstrate tenderness over both the anterior scalene muscle and pectoralis minor muscle. Therefore, blocks are usually performed over both muscles during the same examination. Physical examination is performed after each block so the extent to which each muscle is contributing to the patient's symptoms can be assessed. When tenderness is noted over only one muscle, only that muscle is blocked (injected).

**Pectoralis Minor Muscle Block**. Using ultrasound can help identify the muscle to be blocked. The technique can also be done without ultrasound by localizing the most tender spot over the pectoralis minor muscle, about 4-5 cm (2 inches) below the collarbone. Our preference has been to use short-acting 1% lidocaine as the anesthetic of choice. This is preferred because occasionally lidocaine runs onto some of the nerve branches of the brachial plexus causing increased numbness, tingling, and/or weakness in the upper extremity. Another side effect is some of the lidocaine spreading to affect the eyelid or the voice. By using a short acting drug, these symptoms will last no more than 30 minutes. This occurs in fewer than 5% of patients receiving blocks and in the large majority of those patients, the effect of lidocaine spilling onto nerves is gone in 5 or 10 minutes and the test may then be continued. However, if the effect on the brachial plexus last longer than 10 minutes, the test is of no value and must be repeated at a later date. Lidocaine can leak onto the nerves even when ultrasound identifies the muscle.

The block is performed by injecting 4cc of 1% lidocaine into the pectoralis minor muscle. The 1 and 1/2 inch needle is introduced at a $45^0$ angle, pointing cephalad (towards the head), to avoid entering the chest and causing a pneumothorax (puncturing the pleura and partially collapsing one lung). The lidocaine is spread out over an area approximately 2 cm wide and 1-2 cm deep by injecting small amounts of lidocaine into one spot at a time and repositioning the needle after each small injection. After each repositioning of the needle, the plunger of the syringe is aspirated (pulled back) to assure that the needle tip is not in a blood vessel. If blood is aspirated, the needle is pulled back a few millimeters, moved to a slightly different spot, and re-aspirated to make sure the injection avoids a blood vessel, and the injection then continues. (**Figure 8A**)

An effective block is determined by loss of the tenderness over the injected area of the chest wall (pectoralis minor muscle) within 1-2 minutes. If the patient has no pectoralis minor muscle tenderness on initial physical examination, a pectoralis minor muscle block is not performed.

If there were symptoms of pain and paresthesia at rest, prior to the block, the patient is asked to describe the degree of improvement that has occurred a few minutes after the block. The physical examination is then repeated within a few minutes of completing the block. The positive findings of the provocative maneuvers, tenderness, and Tinel's sign, prior to the muscle block are the baseline from which improvement is measured. A good response to the block is improvement in the majority of positive findings that were present prior to the block. This response is recorded.

If the patient still has residual symptoms after the repeat physical examination is completed, a scalene muscle block is performed while the pectoralis minor muscle block is still in effect. In this way it is possible to assess the role of both the scalene and the pectoralis minor muscles at the same time.

**Anterior Scalene Muscle Block**. The most tender spot over the anterior scalene muscle is determined and the same protocol for the pectoralis minor block is followed for the anterior scalene muscle block. A good block is indicated by loss of tenderness in the injected area. Again, improvement in symptoms is recorded following the block with the patient at rest. The physical examination is repeated after determining that the block was effective, as evidenced by loss of tenderness in the area within 1-2 minutes. As with the pectoralis minor block, a good response is improvement in the majority of positive findings that were present prior to the block. (**Figure 8B**)

FIGURE 8: DIAGNOSTIC MUSCLE BLOCKS: A & B

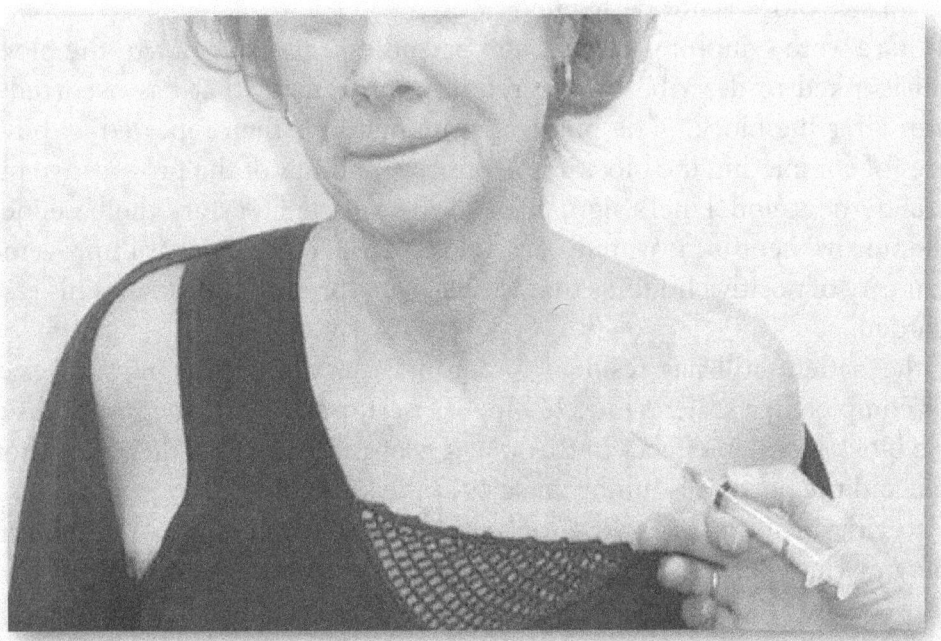

A. Pectoralis minor muscle block: Injection is just below the collarbone.

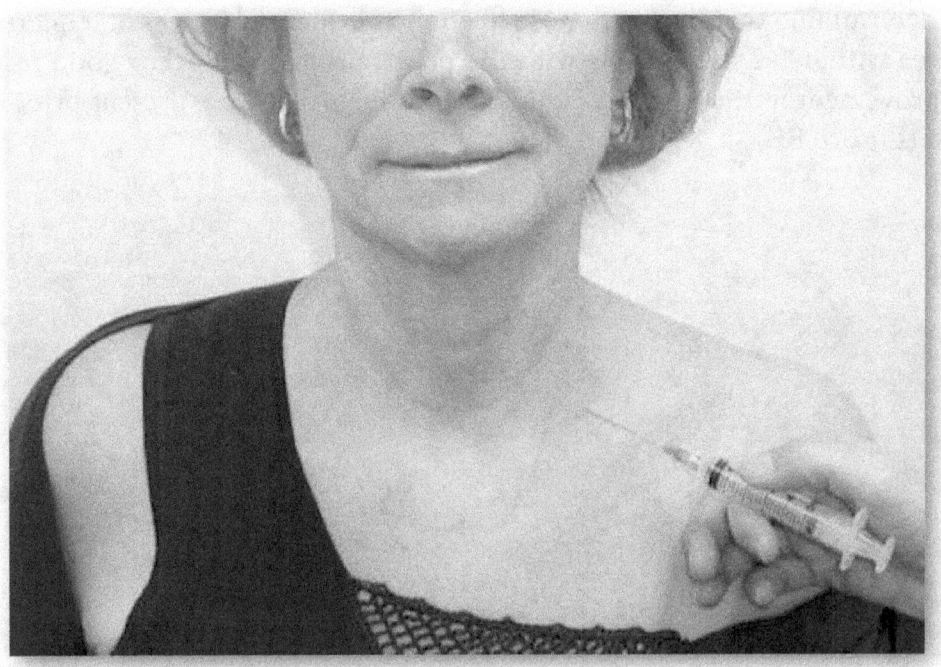

B. Scalene muscle block: Injection is just above the collarbone.

## ELECTRODIAGNOSTIC TESTS.

Nerve testing (electromyography or EMG) can be helpful in a variety of nerve diseases. However, in the past, nerve testing with its many measurements, has seldom been helpful in diagnosing NTOS and NPMS. The exception is the 5% of NTOS patients with congenital cervical ribs, anomalous first ribs, or those with bands arising from a transverse process of C7. In the other 95% of NTOS patients who lacked abnormal ribs or bands, the results of standard EMG studies have usually been normal. However, this is changing.

As an additional part of EMG studies, measurement of the medial antebrachial cutaneous nerve (abbreviated **MAC**) in NTOS patients was first introduced in 1993 by Nishhida et al[11] (**Nishida 1993**). Subsequently, Kothari et al confirmed it in 1998[12] (**Kothari 1998**). In both of these studies, patients had significant symptoms plus other abnormal objective findings.

In 2004, Seror reported that MAC measurements were abnormal in all 16 of 16 patients who had only mild clinical findings (findings on history and physical examination) of NTOS and no objective findings or abnormal ribs.[13] (**Seror 2004**). He described a significant reduction in the amplitude (the height as measured on graph paper or an oscilloscope) of the response to MAC nerve stimulation.

In 2008, Machanic and Sanders reported MAC studies in 41 patients operated upon for NTOS.[14] (**Machanic 2008**) They found not only reduction in amplitude (the magnitude of the response), but also noted reduction in latency (the time required for the stimulus to elicit a response) and slowing of C8 nerve conduction. None of these patients had abnormal ribs, but all had clinical findings supporting a diagnosis of NTOS. 40 of these 41 patients had abnormalities in at least one of the four diagnostic criteria for MAC measurements. All of the patients with good results from surgery who were studied after surgery showed improvement in their MAC measurements.

**MAC and C8 nerve stimulation measurements have become the first consistent objective findings in the diagnosis of either NTOS or NPMS in patients who do not have cervical or anomalous first ribs.**

### Imaging studies

In an earlier era, the only imaging study available was a plain x-ray of the neck. Currently, this is still used as it is the simplest and least expensive way of determining the presence or absence of a cervical or anomalous first rib. (**Figure 4**) However, there are now a variety of other imaging techniques available which can be used to confirm a diagnosis of NTOS or NPMS. While these tests can be helpful, they are usually unnecessary. With a good history, physical xamination, positive response to muscle blocks, and abnormal responses to EMG tests, additional, and more expensive, diagnostic studies are seldim indicated or needed to diagnose NTOS or NPMS.

**Magnetic Resonance Imaging (MRI)** of the brachial plexus can at times show nerve compression, but many times will be normal.[15] **(Bulanger 2013)** The same MRI of the neck, when looking at the cervical spine, can demonstrate bulging discs or spinal or foraminal stenosis (narrowing in the bony canal containing the spinal cord or the holes in the bony spine through which pass the nerves to the arm). **(Figure 9A & B)**. In the future, when MRI can detect muscular scarring, MRI could become more useful. Magnetic Resonance Angiography (MRA) is useful in diagnosing arterial or venous TOS, but is not indicated for neurogenic TOS. Ultrasound and CT scans seldom add to the diagnosis of neurogenic TOS although they may be helpful for arterial or venous TOS.

**Neurography.** This is a technique that can demonstrate displacement or distortion of nerves of the brachial plexus.[16] **(Filler 2009)** This can help confirm a diagnosis of NTOS when severe trauma has occurred. However, like other imaging techniques, when the diagnosis can be confirmed by less expensive methods, neurography is unnecessary.

# FIGURE 9.  MRI OF CERVICAL SPINE: NORMAL  & SPINAL STENOSIS

**A.  Normal Cervical Spine**          **B.  Spinal Stenosis**

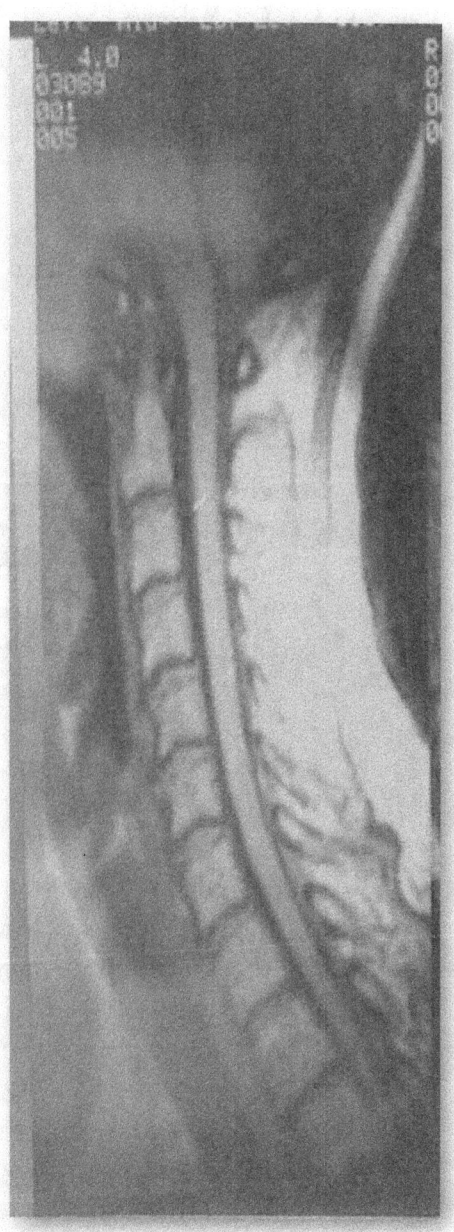

Figure 9:  A.  The spinal cord is the slightly curved solid white column. It is normal. B. Arthritis bony spurs press against the spinal cord as indicated by white arrows.

### Differential and Associated Diagnoses

The association of NTOS and NPMS with other diagnoses is quite common and labeled Double Crush Syndrome.[1] (**Upton 1973**) This indicates that there are at least two areas of nerve compression and sometimes three. Among the diagnoses that can coexist with NTOS and NPMS or must be differentiated from it are: Cervical spine disease, shoulder pathology (disease), ulnar nerve compression at the elbow (also called cuboid tunnel syndrome), carpal tunnel, pronator tunnel, and radial tunnel syndromes. These are listed in **Table 4**.

## TABLE 4

### DIFFERENTIAL AND ASSOCIATED DIAGNOSES (OTHER CONDITIONS THAT CAN PRESENT WITH SIMLAR SYMPTOMS)

1. Cervical spine disease
2. Shoulder pathology (disease)
3. Carpal Tunnel Syndorme (median nerve compression at the wrist)
4. Cuboid Tunnel Syndrome (ulnar nerve compression at the elbow)
5. Pronator Tunnel Syndrome (ulnar nerve compression in inner forearm)
6. Radial Tunnel Syndrome (radial nerve compression in top of forearm)

## TREATMENT OF NTOS

### Indications for treatment

When associated diagnoses exist and conservative treatment has been unsuccessful, it is often difficult to decide on which condition to operate first. In general, the condition bothering the patient most will be treated first. If most symptoms are below the elbow, carpal and cuboid tunnel compression will be treated first. When neck pain, occipital headaches, and shoulder girdle pain predominate, NTOS and NPMS will be treated first. Many times, after one condition has been treated successfully, symptoms from the other conditions may subside to the point that no further treatment is necessary. However, from time to time, a second or even third diagnosis will require surgical treatment at a later time.

The co-existence of NTOS with NPMS is another form of double crush. Depending on responses to diagnostic tests and muscle blocks, it may be decided to treat just one of these first and note the response before treating the second. Since the operation for NPMS is a simple, minimal risk outpatient procedure, pectoralis minor release will be the one performed first as recovery takes less than a week, and patients are usually able to return to work in a few days. If this provides good relief of symptoms, further surgery is avoided. If relief is minimal or only partial, a more extensive operation for NTOS can be performed at a later date.

## CONSERVATIVE TREATMENT

Treatment for NTOS and NPMS is either conservative (non-surgical) or surgical. Conservative therapy is always performed first. Conservative treatment includes altering activity, physical therapy (PT), chiropractic manipulation, osteopathic manipulation, acupuncture, and medication. For patients working on keyboards at computers, creating ergonomic work-stations may prove helpful. Medication includes anti-inflammatory drugs, muscle relaxants, and pain relievers. If all of these fail, and if symptoms are severe enough to interfere with work, recreation, sleep, or activities of daily living, surgery is the next consideration.

### Physical therapy (PT)

NTOS and NPMS are treated together in PT. There are several protocols for PT, including the Edgelow protocol[17] (**Edgelow 2013**), each of which has been effective in some patients. Our preference for therapy includes the modalities listed in **Table 5**.

The stretching exercises should be performed three times a day. Each stretch is held for 15-20 seconds. Each stretch is followed by resting for same length of time. At each stretching session, each stretch is performed three times. Neck stretching includes two separate stretches: rotating the chin over the shoulder is one stretch (**Figure 6A**); tilting the head, ear to shoulder (**Figure 6B**), is the second neck stretch. Both neck stretches should be performed at each session.

Pectoralis minor stretching can be performed in a few different ways: Standing in an open doorway with each hand on the door jam at shoulder height (**Figure 10**) or standing in the corner of a room and placing the hands against each wall at shoulder height. In either position, the upper body falls forward without bending at the waist. Another technique is to place the hand of the involved side against a wall with the elbow bent and rotate the body away from the hand.

Nerve glides are performed by extending the arms $90^0$ to the side with the elbows straight, and bending the wrists back and forth 10-15 times, pointing the fingers upwards (toward the ceiling) then downwards (towards the floor).

Correct posture is holding the spine straight with the head partially held backwards and chin held partially down. The shoulders are in a neutral position, neither hunched forward nor hyperextended backward in a military attention position. (**Figure 11**)

**Abdominal breathing** is performed with the patient lying flat on the floor, preferably without a pillow, but a pillow can be used if necessary. A hand is placed on the abdomen over the belly button. When taking a deep breath in (inspiration), the hand is pushed upwards indicating that the diaphragm is doing the breathing. When blowing out the breath with the diaphragm (expiration), the hand on the belly falls, again indicating that the diaphragm is doing the work. Most of the time, people breath by using their chest wall muscles (between the ribs). When using these muscles (intercostal muscles) to breath, the hand falls with inspiration and rises with expiration.

Therapy initially should be continued for three months. Most modalities, such as stretching, nerve glides, and abdominal breathing, should be performed daily, at home. An important role of the therapist is to instruct patients on how to perform each modality; follow up visits with the patients are to make sure they are performing them correctly. Some modalities require hands on treatment by a therapist, such as dry needling, manual therapy, and passive stretching.

In general, strengthening exercises with therabands and weights or resistance machines, should be avoided. These usually exacerbate symptoms of NTOS and NPMS although they may be helpful for other conditions. Similarly, neck traction is of no help for NTOS or NPMS and may make these conditions worse, while neck traction can be very helpful for cervical spine conditions.

Other forms of conservative treatment, such as heat, massage, acupuncture, and ultrasound often give temporary relief of symptoms. These are often used along with other modalities.

The Feldenkrais Method has been helpful to many patients.[18] (**Buchanan 2001**) Additional forms of conservative therapy are often employed on a trial and error basis, each with occasional success.

Chiropractic therapy has sometimes provided relief of neurogenic symptoms. If chiropractic therapy has not provided some relief within 3 months, other forms of therapy should be sought.

## TABLE 5

Physical Therapy

**A. Preferred Modalities (techniques)**
Neck stretching
Pectoralis minor stretching
Posture correction
Nerve glides
Abdominal breathing (breathing with diaphragm)
Feldenkrais Method

**B. Ineffective modalities for NTOS and NPMS**
Strengthening exercises
Resistance exercises
Therabands
Neck traction

# FIG 10. PECTORALIS MINOR MUSCLE STRETCH IN OPEN DOORWAY

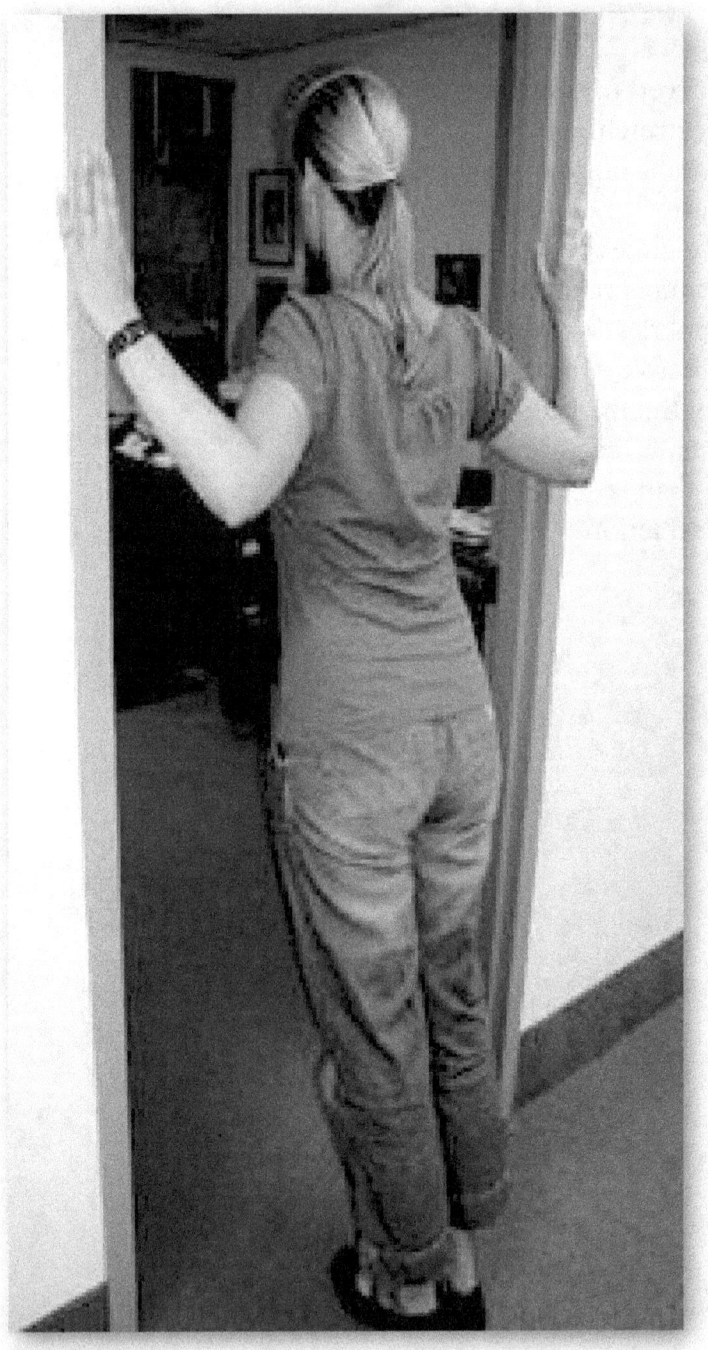

Figure 10: With hands on the door jam, the body leans forward with knees straight.

## FIGURE 11: CORRECT POSTURE

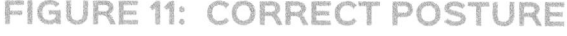

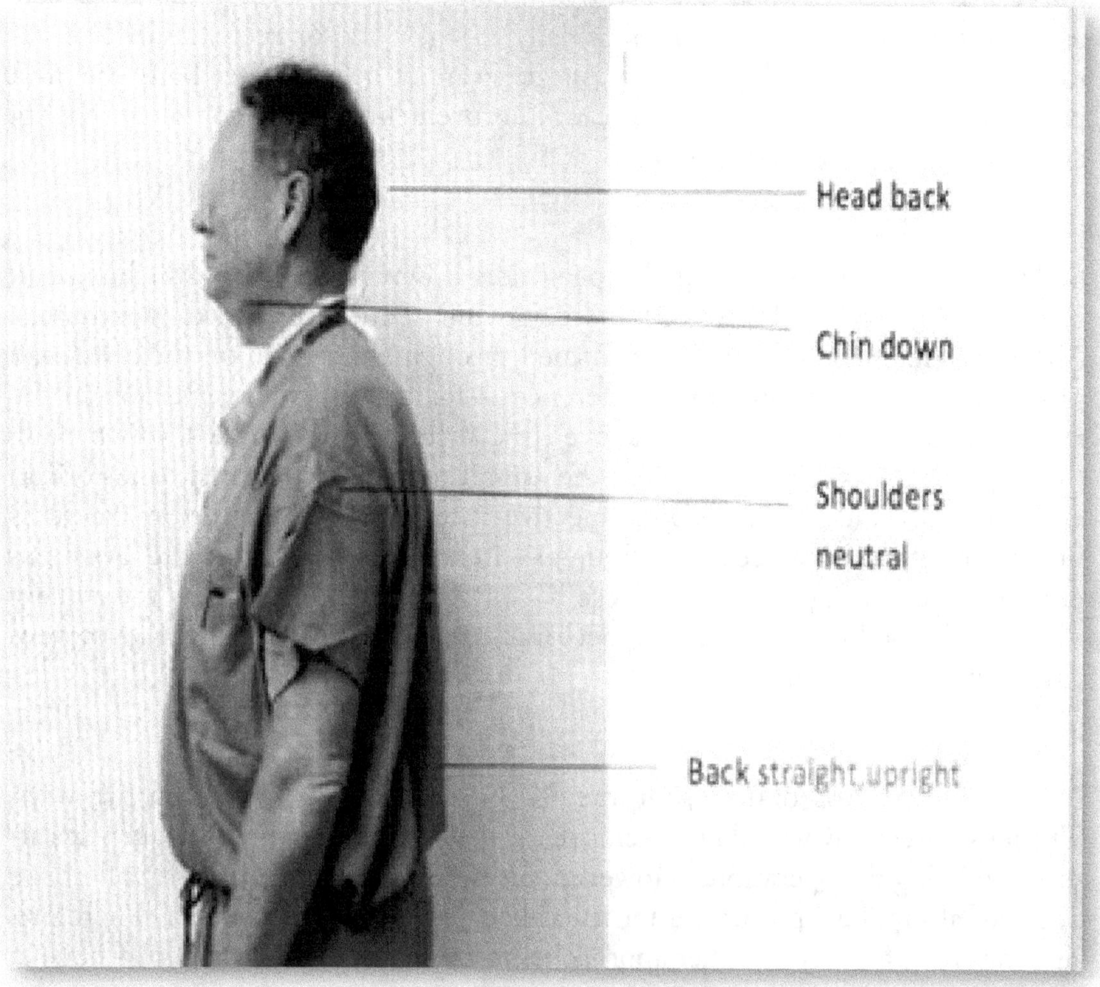

Head back

Chin down

Shoulders neutral

Back straight, upright

Figure 11: Correct posture. Head back; Chin down; shoulders neutral, neither held forward nor backward.

## SURGICAL TREATMENT

Surgery is indicated when conservative therapy fails and symptoms are severe enough to interfere with activities of daily living, work, or recreation. The patient must realize that the results of surgery cannot be guaranteed and for most patients, a good result means significant improvement, but not complete relief of every symptom under all conditions.

### Neurogenic Pectoralis Minor Syndrome

Surgery for NPMS is cutting the pectoralis minor at its bony attachment to the coracoid process (**Figure 2**) and removing about one inch of the muscle. Although the operation can be performed through an incision on the chest wall just below the collarbone, our preference is for a transaxillary incision in the front portion of the armpit, just above the hairline.[19] (**Sanders 2010**) Through this approach, it is easier to explore the armpit to severe thickened bands of clavipectoral fascia (a thin layer of connective tissue covering the major structures in the armpit) and the occasional Langer's arch which arises from the latissimus dorsi muscle.[20] (**Magee 2012**) These bands of tissue can compress the axillary nerves and blood vessels in the subpectoral space. (**Page 52, Technique of pectoralis minor tenotomy**)

### Neurogenic Thoracic Outlet Syndrome

Neurogenic thoracic outlet syndrome (NTOS) can be approached in five ways. The most direct way would be to remove the collarbone and put it back in place after completing the operation. However, this is rarely done because the collarbone does not always heal properly after it has been temporarily removed. Therefore, surgeons have found four other approaches to the area that leave the collarbone in tact.

**Approaches to the thoracic outlet**. The four avenues through which to reach the thoracic outlet area by leaving the clavicle alone are:

1. Through the armpit (axilla), the transaxillary approach;
2. above the collarbone, the supraclavicular approach;
3. below the collarbone, the infraclavicular approach; or
4. behind the collarbone through the back, using an incision along the scapula, the posterior approach.

The last two approaches, 3 and 4, are seldom used. The posterior approach is avoided, if possible, because it requires cutting some of the back muscles near the shoulder blade. This occasionally results in postoperative back pain which can be debilitating and is very hard to treat. The exposure of the brachial plexus is from behind and is not as good as the supraclavicular approach. The posterior approach is used primarily for reoperations when other approaches have failed. Going through the posterior route avoids the scar tissue that will be found by re-operating through routes previously used.

The infraclavicular approach is used for reaching the anterior portion of the rib. It can be combined with a supraclavicular approach to achieve "complete" removal of the first rib, a procedure called "over and under"[21] (**Robicsek 1997**) or the paraclavicular approach. [22] (**Thompson 1992**) However, it should be pointed out that even though the supraclavicular approach cannot reach the anterior portion of the first rib, experience has shown that it is seldom necessary to remove the anterior rib portion when treating NTOS alone. On the other hand, when treating VTOS, the anterior portion of the rib must be removed and the infraclavicular approach is selected if repair of the subclavian vein is anticipated. The transaxillary approach is our practice for VTOS when only first rib resection and complete freeing of the subclavian vein is planned.

The supraclavicular and transaxillary routes are the most popular routes to decompress the thoracic outlet for NTOS. The two different approaches, through the neck or through the armpit, relieve the same symptoms. As of this writing, there is no significance difference in long-term results between the two operations.[23] (**Sanders, Pearce 1989**)

**The supraclavicular approach** is through an incision at the base of the neck, just above the collarbone. It provides the best exposure of the scalene triangle, its muscles, and the brachial plexus. Through this incision the entire anterior and middle scalene muscles can be removed as well as cervical ribs and the portion of the first rib near the nerves. With this exposure one can determine whether the first rib can be left in tact or removed. This is the only approach that permits complete removal of scar tissue from all of the nerve roots going to the arm. In ATOS, this approach permits removing abnormal ribs and also repairing or replacing the subclavian artery. The primary disadvantage of the supraclavicular approach is it is accompanied by a little higher incidence of injury to the phrenic and long thoracic nerves and the lymphatic ducts (left side only). The supraclavicular approach should not be used in VTOS, unless it is accompanied by an infraclavicular incision (the paraclavicular approach[22] Thompson) to remove the anterior portion of the rib and decompression of the subclavian vein.

**The transaxillary approach,** through the armpit, is the best approach for freeing compressive structures from around the subclavian vein, including the anterior part of the first rib. This approach is also convenient for performing, with just one incision, pectoralis minor tenotomy, and then proceeding deeper to remove the first rib. The primary disadvantages of the transaxillary route are that exposure is more difficult and it is harder to remove the entire posterior portion of the rib. In addition, because of the limited exposure, it is more complicated to teach trainees how to perform this operation. The advantages and disadvantages of the two preferred approaches are listed in **Table 6.**

## TABLE 6

## ADVANTAGES & DISADVANTAGES OF TRANSAXILLARY AND SUPRACLAVICULAR APPROACHES

### TRANSAXILLARY APPROACH

#### Advantages

1. Best approach for removal of front portion of the first rib
2. Probably an easier way to remove the middle portion of the first rib
3. Best approach for freeing the subclavain vein in Venous TOS
4. Less chance of phrenic nerve injury
5. Dissection is limited to just the lower nerves, not the entire brachial plexus
6. Rarely encounter lymphatics compared to the supraclavicular approach

#### Disadvantages

1. Harder to remove the back part of the rib than the supraclavicular approach
2. More likely to enter the chest space than the supraclavicular approach
3. Exposure is more difficult and a harder approach to teach to others
4. Cannot repair or replace the subclavian artery through this route for arterial TOS
5. Harder to repair an injury in the subclavian artery or vein through this route

# SUPRACLAVICULAR APPROACH

## Advantages

1. Can remove most or all of the anterior and middle scalene muscles
2. Better exposure of all nerves and easier to identify congenital bands
3. Can elect to remove or leave in place the first rib as the first rib is not the primary source of the pathology (disease)
4. It is easier to evaluate and remove most cervical ribs through this approach
5. In arterial TOS, the subclavian artery can be repaired or replaced through the neck
6. Can perform complete neurolysis (removal of scar tissue) of all five nerve roots and three trunks
7. Easier to remove the posterior first rib close to the transverse process of the spine

## Disadvantages

1. Can't remove the anterior part of the first rib
2. More likely to injure the phrenic and long thoracic nerves than the transaxillary approach
3. Greater risk of lymphatic leakage (on the left side only) than the trans-axillary approach

**Technique of supraclavicular approach.** The special instruments are seen in **Figure 12**. Details of this technique were most recently described in 2015.[24] (**Sanders 2015**)

The patient is anesthetized and a breathing tube is placed in the windpipe. The skin incision is 5-7 cm long and lies just above and parallel to the collarbone. This transverse incision is used because it heals with minimal scarring and the scar blends in with natural skin lines in the neck. Because the rest of the operation requires a vertical exposure, the skin is under-cut by raising upper and lower skin flaps. The sternocleidomastoid muscle (SCM) is mobilized on its lateral (outside) edge and retracted medially (toward the midline). While older descriptions of this operation describe cutting the lateral half of the SCM muscle, this is unnecessary and can leave an undesired permanent depression on the side of the neck. By mobilizing the lateral edge of the SCM and retracting (pulling back) the muscle, exposure is just as good as cutting the muscle and a depression is avoided.

A self-retaining retractor (Mini-Omintract[R]) is attached to the operating table to provide excellent vision of the deep structures. The omohyoid muscle is removed and the scalene fat pad is opened vertically. The nerves to the arm (the brachial plexus) are identified and the individual nerve roots are freed of scar tissue. (**Figure 13A-L**) It is unnecessary to initially identify the phrenic nerve. In most cases, the phrenic nerve is best sought **after** the brachial plexus has first been dissected.

FIGURE 12: INSTRUMENTS

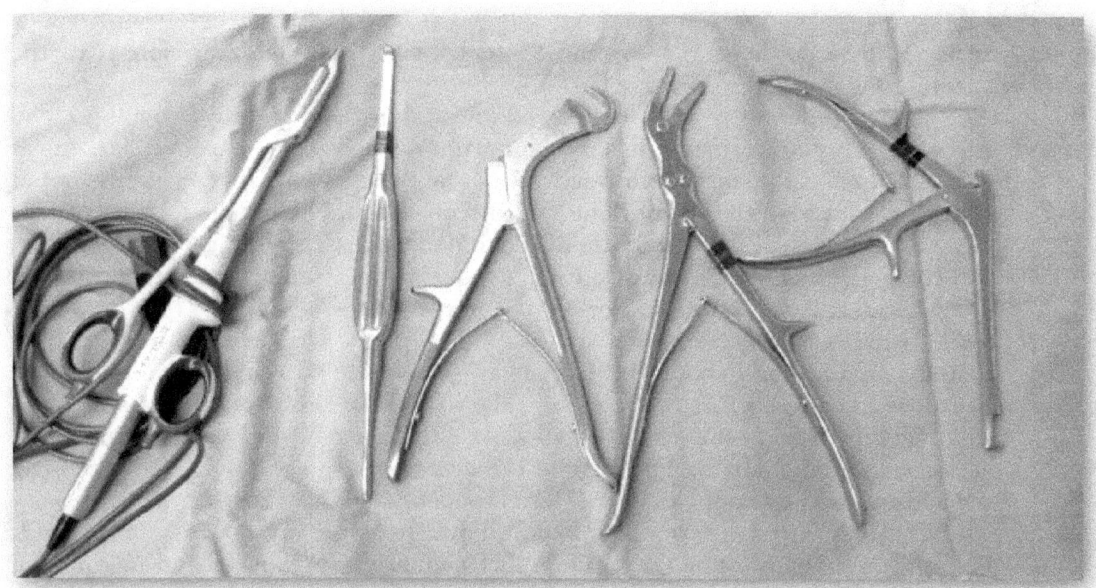

Figure 12: Instruments for supraclavicular rib resection: From left to right, harmonic scalpel, Overholt #1 periosteal elevator, Shoemaker rib cutter, infraclavicular rib cutter (Pilling), and Raney rongeur.

Figure 13: Technique of supraclavicular scalenectomy and first rib resection. Drawings by artist Amalia Christman.

A. Incision, 1-2 cm above clavicle and 5-7 cm long. This neck incision gives the smallest and most pleasing scar.

B. The skin is undercut to raise upper and lower skin flaps thereby providing good exposure. This converts the field of vision from a transverse one to a vertical one as the muscles and the nerves run vertically. The figure shows dissecting the upper skin flap just above the sternocleidomastoid muscle and below the fat beneath the platysma muscle. SCM = sternocleidomastoid muscle which has just been exposed.

C. A retractor pulls the SCM muscle back, exposing a layer of fat, the scalene fat pad. The fat pad must be divided to expose the nerves to the arm.

D. The C5 nerve root is freed of scar tissue. This is the first of the 5 nerves going to the arm and hand that will be freed of scar tissue to relieve symptoms. C5 is exposed and two of its branches are identified, the suprascapular nerve to the shoulder blade and sometimes a branch to the phrenic nerve (also called the accessory phrenic nerve). The edge of the anterior scalene muscle (ASM) may be seen. The middle scalene muscle (MSM) is also partially exposed.

E. The C5, C6, C7, and C8, are dissected free of scar tissue. The last nerve root, T1, lies under C8 and is found later. The subclavian artery is exposed and surrounded with a soft plastic loop to help move it to the side when needed.

F. The anterior scalene muscle (ASM) is divided near its first rib attachment with a harmonic scalpel.

# FIGURE 13: TECHNIQUE OF SUPRACLAVICULAR DECOMPRESSION

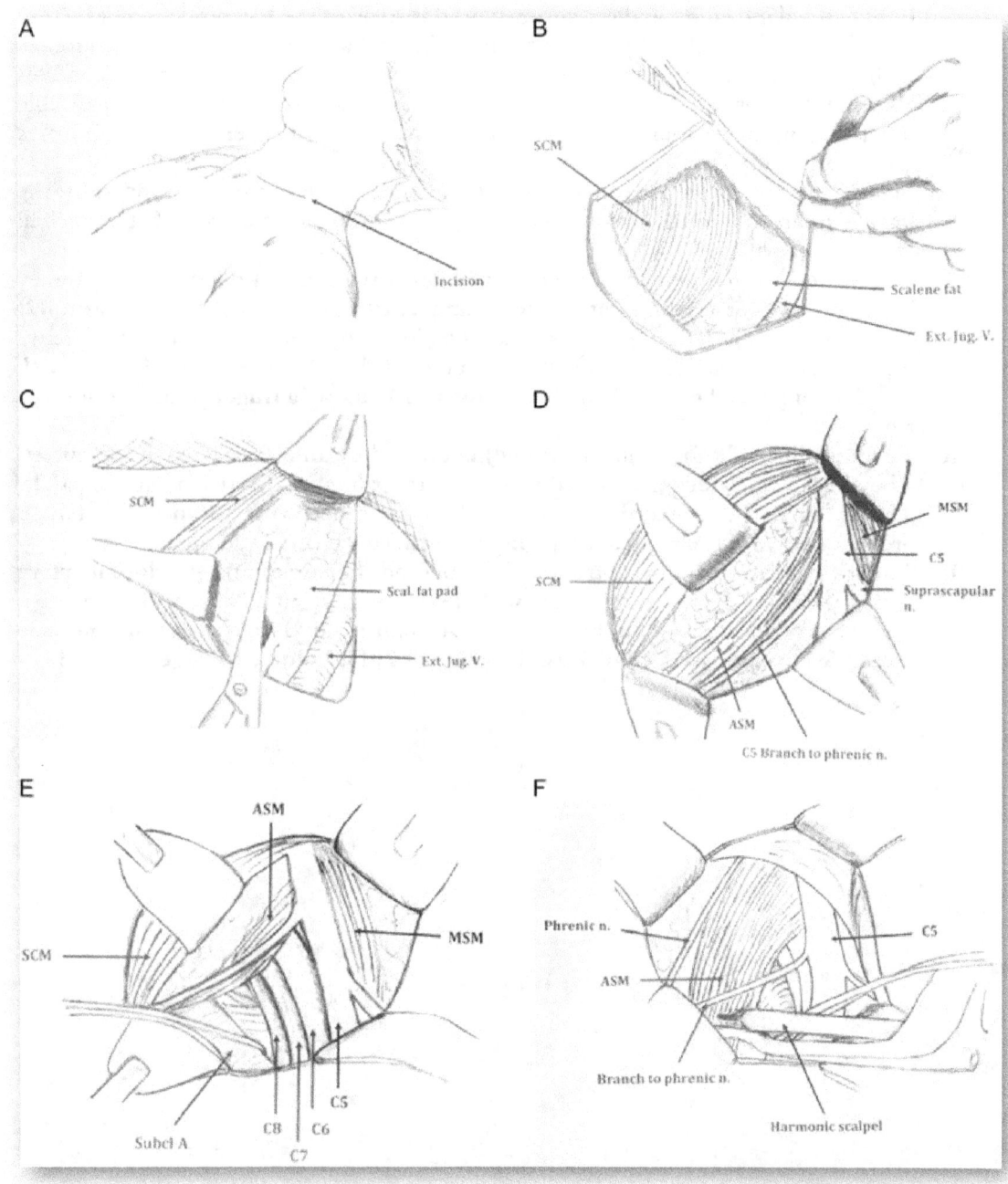

Figure 13: Continued

G. The freed lower end of ASM is grasped with a clamp, elevated, and the upper end of ASM is divided above the C5 nerve root with a harmonic scalpel. If space is too tight, a bipolar cautery and scissors are used instead of the harmonic scalpel. Care is taken to protect the phrenic nerve from being handled, irritated, or stretched. If this is injured, shortness of breath can occur because one phrenic nerve controls about 20% of breathing. Even if injured, most patients have little or no trouble breathing but may experience some shortness of breath on exertion. Such injuries are usually temporary.

H. Identifying the branches of the long thoracic nerve that are surrounded by the muscle fibers. Note the plastic vessel loop surrounding the nerves of the brachial plexus.

I. The posterior part(the neck) of the first rib, near the spine, is divided with a Raney rongeur. If there is enough room, the Shumaker rib cutter may be used. (Figure 12)

J. One centimeter of first rib has been excised (cut away) and a finger frees the pleura (the covering of the lung) from the underside of the rib. The rib is elevated with the right angle end of a periosteal elevator which allows a finger to get behind the rib.

K. The anterior end of the rib (front end) is divided by an infraclavicular rib cutter. The subclavian artery is elevated to permit the rib cutter to reach the rib safely. The stump of the remaining anterior rib is smoothed with a Raney rongeur to prevent the tip of the rib from injuring the subclavian artery lying above it.

L. The divided rib section is extracted from behind the nerves and subclavian artery with a Kocher clamp. Reprinted with permission from Elsiever. Sanders RJ, Annest SJ. Technique of Supraclavicular Decompression for Neurogenic Thoracic Outlet Syndrome. Journal of Vascular Surgery 2015; Volume 61:pages 821-825.[25]

# FIGURE 13: TECHNIQUE OF SUPRACLAVICULAR DECOMPRESSION, CONT.

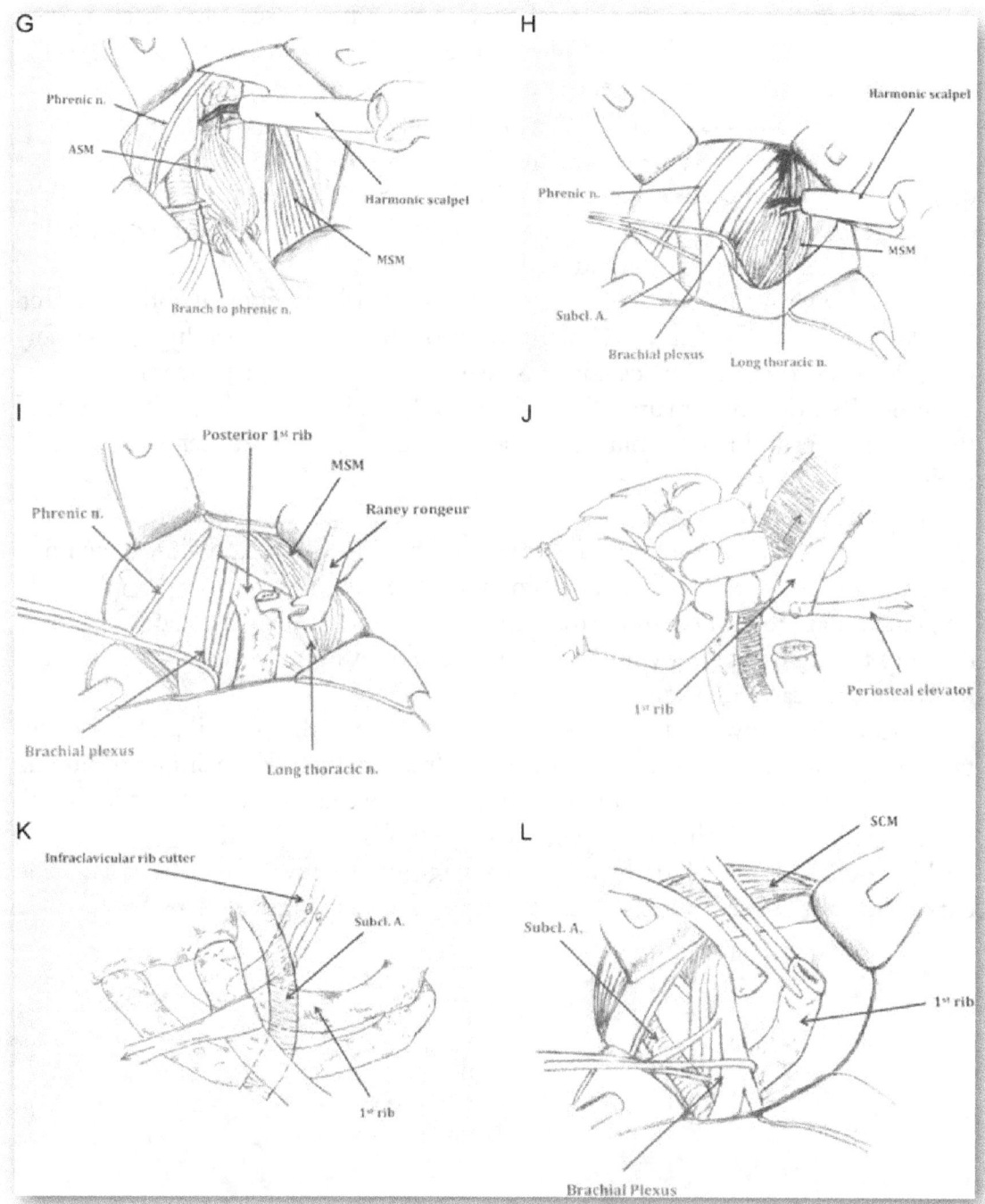

After finding C5, a small branch arising on its inner side should be sought, as it is the C5 contribution to the phrenic nerve, sometimes called the accessory phrenic. When present, this branch is protected as C6 and C7 are dissected free. C8 and T1 may be freed next, or if the lateral edge of the anterior scalene muscle is seen to be covering the lower brachial plexus, the anterior scalene muscle is dissected and the main phrenic nerve identified, usually on the medial (inner) edge of the anterior scalene muscle. In 13% of patients, the phrenic nerve lies on the lateral (outer) side of the anterior scalene muscle.[25] **(Sanders, Roos 1989)** This makes dissection difficult because this nerve must be preserved and it lies in the middle of the operative field. When necessary, a soft plastic vessel loop is carefully used to move the phrenic gently to the side.

The anterior scalene muscle is divided at its first rib attachment and is elevated with a clamp, freed from its attachments to the spine and divided as high as is safely possible. With the anterior scalene muscle gone, exposure of the lower nerve roots is easier. Removal of remaining scar tissue and bands is completed from around the nerve roots and trunks, but the loose connective tissue between the nerves is left alone.

The middle scalene muscle is now dissected lateral to C5. Because the C5 and C6 branches of the long thoracic nerve lie in the midst of the middle scalene muscle, dissection is by a few fibers at a time until the long thoracic nerve and two of its branches are identified and preserved. The middle scalene muscle is dissected down to the first rib, removing enough fibers so that none are left contacting the nerves of the brachial plexus.

A decision is now made whether or not to remove the first rib. If the lower trunk of the brachial plexus is within 1-2 mm (millimeters) of touching the rib, the rib is removed. If there is 2 mm or more space between the nerve and rib, the rib can be left in tact. With experience, it has been observed that first ribs which are fairly straight and lie high in the neck usually require removal; first ribs with a wide curve, the ones harder to excise, can be left untouched. **(Figure 14A&B)**

FIGURE 14 A

CURVED FIRST RIB

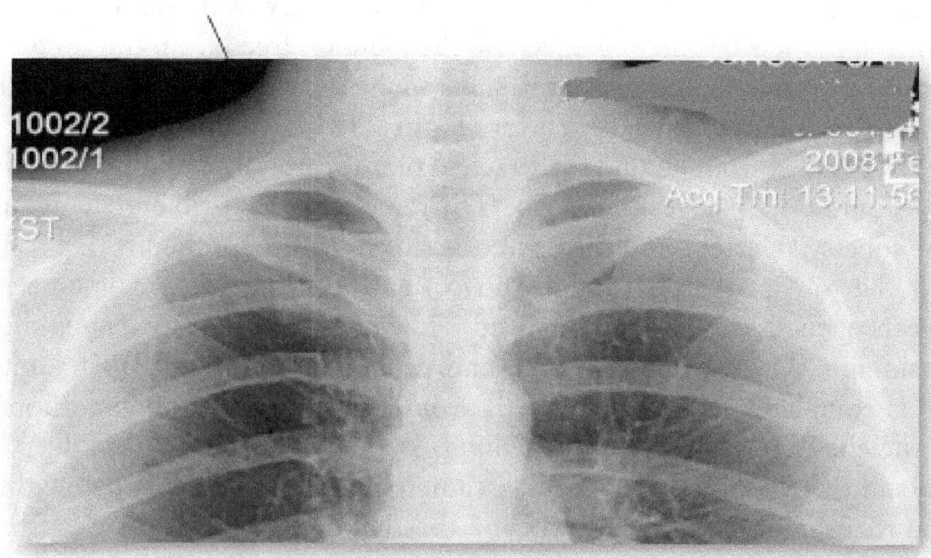

FIGURE 14 B

STRAIGHT FIRST RIB

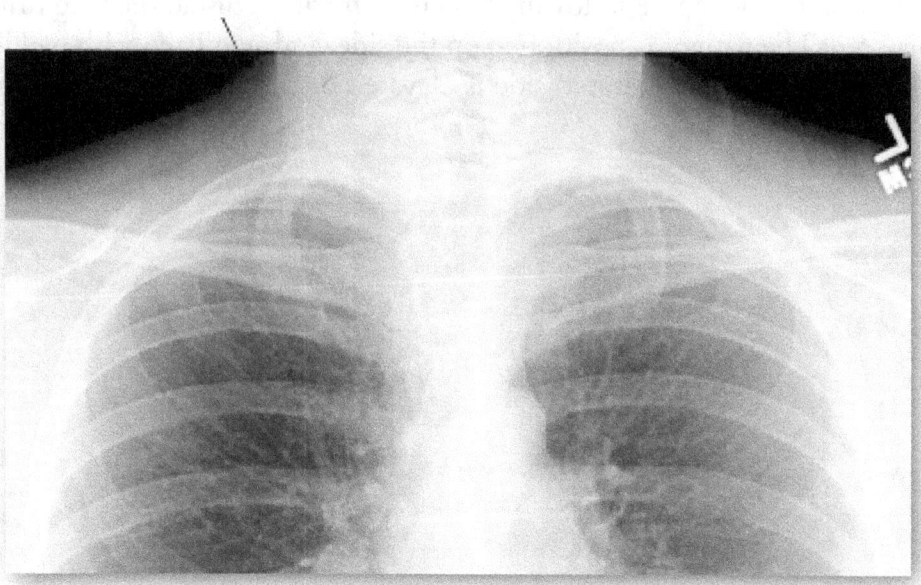

Figure 14: X-ray of first rib helps decide whether or not to remove the rib: A. Curved first rib can usually be left in place; B. Straight first rib usually requires removal.

First rib resection begins by excising enough middle scalene muscle to expose the neck of the rib. The intercostal muscles (between ribs) are detached and the medial (inner) rib edge is freed with a periosteal elevator (special instrument, **Figure 12**) which also frees the brachial plexus and subclavian artery from the rib. The posterior portion of the rib is then divided and the pleura is freed from the rib by finger dissection. Carefully pulling back the subclavian artery, the anterior end of the rib is cut with an infraclavicular rib cutter (**Figure 12**). The divided piece of rib is carefully extracted from behind the brachial plexus carefully avoiding scraping the nerves with the sharp edges of the rib. The remaining front rib end, lying just below the subclavian artery, and the posterior rib end, are smoothed with a rongeur.

Whether or not the pleura (lung space) has been opened, we assume it may have been opened even if not visualized. The anesthesiologist expands the lung and maintains the patient in positive end expiratory pressure (PEEP) until the wound is completely closed. This will avoid a postoperative pneumothorax (air inside the chest collapsing part of the lung). A suction drain is placed deep in the wound and the wound closed. A small catheter can be placed just below the skin incision for administration of a local anesthesthetic for 24 to 48 hours after ssurgery for pain control.

## TRANSAXILLARY APPROACH

**Technique of transaxillary first rib resection.** The patient is anesthetized and a tube placed in the windpipe following which no further muscle relaxing drugs are administered. The patient is positioned on the side, and stabilized with padded hip clamps. The arm of the operated side is elevated on a special, sterile arm holder. (**Figure 15**)

FIGURE 15 B:  TABLE MOUNTED ARM HOLDER

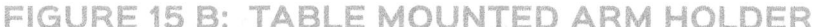

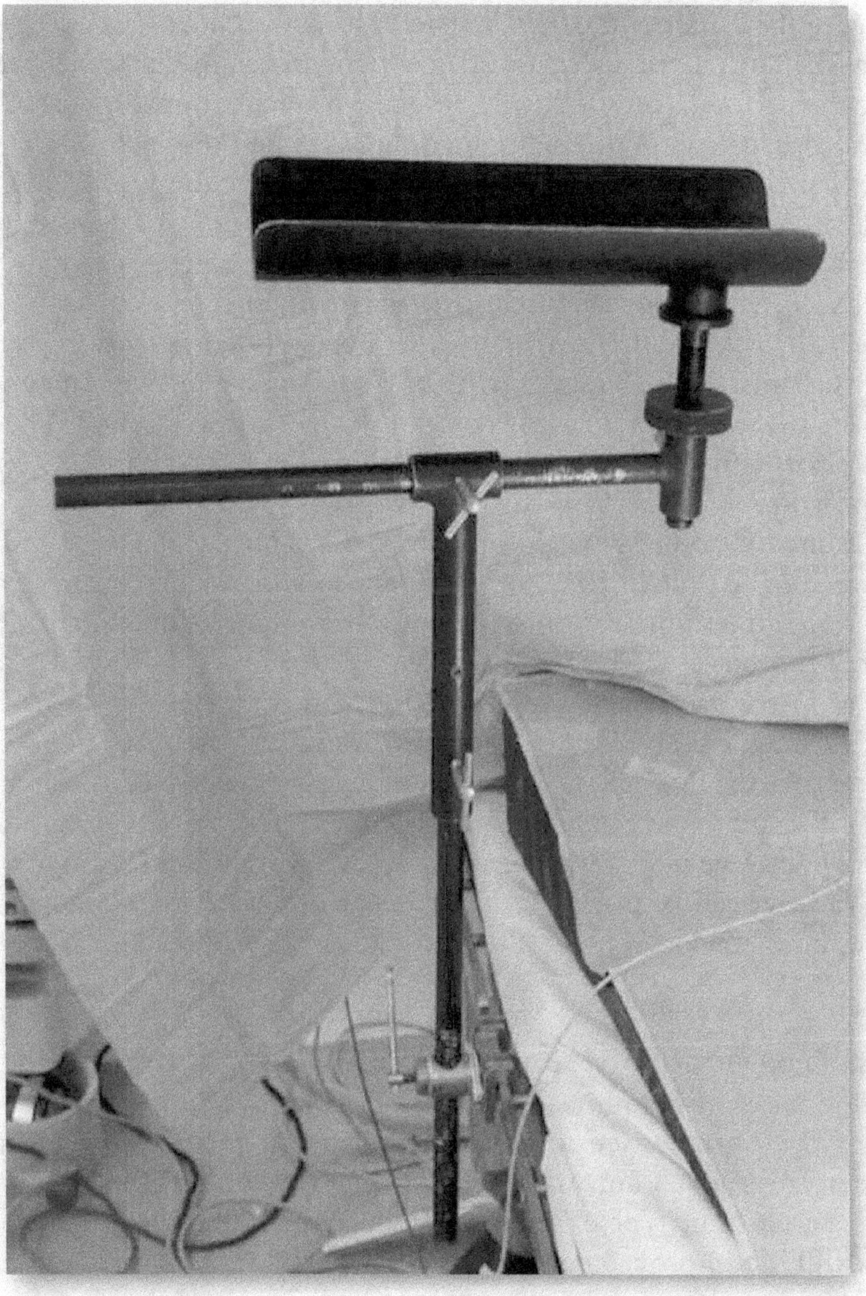

Figure 15:  Sterile adjustable arm holder, designed by Dr. James Sessions and Dr. David Roos, attaches to the table.

A 5-7 cm transverse incision is made in the armpit. Subcuateous tissue is divided, trying to identify and preserve the 2nd intercostal brachial cutaneous nerve. If the nerve lies in the center of the field, the nerve is divided because an over-stretched nerve causes much more discomfort than a numb patch of skin under the arm. If dividing the pectoralis minor muscle has been planned, the muscle is now identified, divided, and 2 cm of pectoralis minor muscle is cut out.

The first rib is now sought, by going down to the chest wall and identifying the first rib by its position under the subclavian vein. The intercostal muscles are divided and the inner and outer edges of the first rib completely freed. The middle and anterior scalene muscles are each divided as far away from the rib as possible. The center portion of the rib is divided as far posterior and anterior as safety permits. The divided section of rib is removed. The remaining anterior rib stump is shortened to the costal cartilage with rongeurs. The remaining posterior stump is the harder one to visualize but is carefully shortened using special protection of the lower nerve trunk. The goal is to leave a posterior rib stump nottoo near the lower nerve. The subclavian artery and vein are now cleared of all remaining anterior scalene muscle attachments, allowing the muscle it to retract upwards, into the neck, to remove as much tension as possible from the nerves to the arm.

Just as in the supraclavicular approach, whether or not the pleura has been opened, we assume it may have been opened even if not visualized. The anesthesiologist expands the lung and maintains the patient in positive end expiratory pressure (PEEP) until the wound is completely closed. This will avoid a postoperative pneumothorax. A suction drain is placed deep in the wound and the incision closed. A small catheter can be placed in the subcutaneous space for administration of a local anesthesthetic for 24 hours after surgery for pain control.

## RESULTS OF TREATMENT FOR NTOS

**Results of conservative treatment** depend on how soon treatment begins following the onset of symptoms. Patients who begin treatment within the first month or two of the onset of symptoms have very good results, regardless of the type of treatment. This is because the majority of NTOS patients develop symptoms after some type of injury. Particularly if the trauma was acute, most patients will see improvement within the first few months without any treatment. Therefore, if treatment is started in the first few weeks after an accident, it is impossible to know if that patient is improving because of the treatment or because of the passage of time and nature's normal healing. On the other hand, if treatment doesn't begin until months or years after symptoms began, the success rate decreases significantly.

If symptoms continue after several months of physical therapy, the options patients have are to continue to live with the symptoms and use home exercises and pain management or consider surgery, where the results cannot be guaranteed. In this situation, if the symptoms are mild, the majority of patients elect to continue to live with the symptoms.

If symptoms are severe, but show some improvement after three months of physical therapy, the therapy is continued until symptoms either improve significantly or plateau. At that point many patients will consider surgery.

If symptoms are severe and show no improvement after three months of appropriate therapy, chances are small that continuing therapy will lead to improvement. At that point the options available are to either continue with more therapy, seek another diagnosis, or consider surgery. Some patients will elect to continue trying non-surgical therapy while others will elect the surgical option.

**Results of surgery for NTOS** vary amongst the many reports in the surgical literature as criteria for evaluating success differ across the world. There are now three or four questionnaires that some medical centers use to help patients describe their symptoms before and after surgery. These can be helpful, but it must be realized that data from patients describing their symptoms are subjective (relying on the patient) and not objective (a test not relying on the patient's description). In general, we have found that asking patients to simply state how much improvement they notice after surgery compared to before surgery is just as reliable as burdensome questionnaires. We essentially want to know first, if the operation failed to provide any improvement. If there is improvement, is it fair, good, or excellent.

The other factor in evaluating results is time. It has been well established that many patients experience significant improvement in the first 3 months following surgery. However, when they return to their preoperative occupation, and over the next 24 months, recurrent symptoms will appear in about 15% of those patients. At least half of the recurrences appear within six months of surgery and 80% are present by two years.[23] (**Sanders 1989**) This must be considered when looking at success rates.

The failure rate of surgery for thoracic outlet syndrome is about the same for either the supraclavicular or transaxillary approach. If there has been no recurrence in the first 24 months after surgery, the chance of recurrence in the next 10-15 years is less than 5%.[23] (**Sanders 1989**) In the same study, the overall success rate was about 75% at 2 years. Since that study was published, surgical techniques have changed only slightly. Statistics are a little better, but are hard to compare because long term results over 10 to 15 years seldom have been published. Although this study was reported in 1989, no other reliable, similar study has been reported showing anything different where both approaches were performed by the same surgeons.

Recurrent or persistent symptoms occur in at least 20% of the patients operated on for NTOS. The symptoms and physical findings are similar to the original symptoms and findings. Diagnostic tests are available but should first be directed towards looking for other causes. If treatable conditions are found in the cervical spine, elbow, wrist, or shoulder, these should be treated first. Evaluation for NPMS should also be performed. If NPMS is present, it should be treated next. If pectoralis minor muscle stretching is unsuccessful, surgical pectoralis minor tenotomy should be considered.[26,27] (**Johanson 2004, Sanders 2011**,) This is a minimal risk outpatient procedure which can reduce symptoms significantly.

If pectoralis minor release does not provide adequate relief, reoperation for NTOS can be performed. The choice of procedure depends upon what was done at previous operations.

1. If the first procedure was transaxillary first rib resection, reoperation is supraclavicular scalenectomy and brachial plexus neurolysis (removal of scar tissue). If there is a long posterior stump of the first rib, it should be shortened, either via the neck or the armpit.
2. If the first procedure was supraclavicular scalenectomy, reoperation is transaxillary first rib resection with or without supraclavicular neurolysis.
3. If the first operation was supraclavicular scalenectomy and first rib resection, reoperation is supraclavicular neurolysis.
4. If the above procedures have all been done and have failed, a last resort procedure is neurolysis plus covering the brachial plexus with a flap of latissimus dorsi muscle. This is an extensive procedure requiring several months for total recovery. The results of this procedure have not yet been reported in the surgical literature.[28] (**Annest 2013**)

# Neurogenic Pectoralis Minor Syndrome: NPMS Alone

The majority of patients with NPMS also have NTOS. Most of the time the two are treated simultaneously. However, it is important to recognize each condition separately, particularly if NPMS is the predominate diagnosis. This is an example of a double crush phenomenon[1](**Upton 1973**) where treating just one of the diagnoses may reduce symptoms enough so that treating the second diagnosis is unnecessary.

## SYMPTOMS

In some patients NPMS is the only diagnosis. Paying close attention to the symptoms and physical findings can make the diagnosis. Symptoms of pain or tenderness in the anterior chest wall and arm pit are usually the chief complaint. Pain over the trapezius muscle (above the shoulder blade) and numbness and tingling in the hand are other frequent symptoms. When these symptoms occur on the left side, particularly the left chest pain, patients may be suspected of having a heart attack. If seen in an emergency room, these symptoms can lead to a complete evaluation for heart disease, including heart catheterization and coronary artery angiograms. When this occurs, and the heart evaluation is completely normal, consideration should be given to a diagnosis of neurogenic pectoralis minor syndrome (NPMS).

## PHYSICAL EXAMINATION

Significant physical findings are tenderness below the collarbone, over the pectoralis minor muscle, and in the armpit. The upper limb tension test is usually positive. (**Figure 5**) Abducting the arm to 90 degrees in external rotation, the elevated arm stress test (**Figure 7**), may be mildly positive as well.[19,29] (**Sanders 2010, Sanders 2007**)

## ETIOLOGY (CAUSE)

Isolated NPMS is usually seen in teenagers or young adults who participate in competitive sports. The sports are those that require repetitive movements of the upper extremities above shoulder level, such as swimming, throwing baseballs or footballs, playing volleyball, and weight lifting. These sports have in common pulling the shoulder blade (scapula) backward with each arm motion. This stretches the pectoralis minor muscle which inserts into the coracoid process, a part of the scapula. The first symptoms may be chest pain or numbness and tingling in the hand.

Many of these patients also have mild symptoms of NTOS, brought about by hyperextension of their neck while they are performing their sport. Therefore, it is not unusual to find these patients being diagnosed first as having NTOS. It is only on a detailed history and physical examination that the diagnosis of NPMS is considered along with the diagnosis of NTOS. In such situation, the response to muscle blocks will demonstrate if the diagnosis of NPMS predominates.

The importance of recognizing NPMS in children was revealed in a study of the results of surgery for NTOS and NPMS in children. Having become aware of NPMS in 2005, a study was made of the results of surgery from 2000 to 2011, and the results were separated into two time periods, between 2000 and 2005, before learning about NPMS, and between 2006 and 2011, after learning about NPMS. In the first five years, all of the operations were thoracic outlet decompression procedures. In the next 5 years, after becoming aware of NPMS, 80% of the operations were pectoralis minor decompression alone while only 20% were thoracic outlet procedures. The conclusion from this analysis was that in the first 5 years a number of thoracic outlet procedures probably should have been pectoralis minor tenotomy.[30] (**Sanders 2013**)

## DIAGNOSTIC TESTS

**Pectoralis minor muscle block**. The block was described earlier in the previous section (**Page 20**). A good response to the block is strong evidence to support the diagnosis of NPMS. In most patients with NPMS alone, most symptoms at rest and findings on repeat physical examination return to normal after the pectoralis minor block. When this occurs, no further block is needed. If some symptoms and positive physical findings remain, a scalene muscle block is performed. If this second block relieves the rest of the symptoms and findings, a diagnosis of both NPMS and NTOS is made. If the patient's relief of symptoms was much greater with the pectoralis minor block, pectoralis minor decompression alone is considered. In such patients the residual symptoms of NTOS can often be ignored or tolerated. If symptoms are significant, thoracic outlet decompression can always be performed at a later date.

**Electrodiagnostic study**. The one objective diagnostic test that has usually been positive is measurement of the medial antebrachial sensory cutaneous nerve.[14](**Machanic 2008**) A positive response is indicative of brachial plexus compression but it cannot separate the thoracic outlet from the pectoralis minor area. However, putting the results together with the clinical picture and the response to the muscle blocks, will help guide the therapeutic decision.

## TREATMENT

**Physical therapy** is always the first approach. For NPMS the therapy is pectoralis minor muscle stretching (**Figure 9**). If performed when symptoms are only a few months old the success rate is quite high. However, if there is no improvement with three months of therapy, surgery is considered.

**Surgery for NPMS** is cutting the pectoralis minor muscle, a minimal risk, outpatient surgical procedure. In experienced hands, the procedure often takes no more than 20 minutes. Recovery time is a few days and complications are rare. The operation can be performed through an incision in the armpit or an incision on the chest wall just below the collarbone. Our preference is a transaxillary incision in the front portion of the armpit, just above the hairline.[19] (**Sanders 2010**)

**Technique of pectoralis minor tenotomy**: A 4-7 cm transverse incision is made 1 cm above the bottom of the axillary hairline beginning in the front of the armpit. The pectoralis minor muscle is identified by its attachment to the coracoid process. Occasionally it is fused to the pectoralis major muscle and must be separated. The pectoralis major muscle is pulled out of the way and the pectoralis minor muscle is divided at its attachment to the shoulder blade (the coracoid process) and 2 cm of pectoralis minor muscle is cut out with a Harmonic scalpel. It is important to avoid the pectoral nerve branches which usually lie about 3 cm from the coracoid and penetrate the pectoralis minor muscle en route to the pectoralis major muscle. Any bands of clavipectoral fascia and the occasional Langer's arch muscle fibers[20] (**Mcgee 2012**) are also removed leaving nothing tight that can compress the nerves or blood vessels that lie under thepectoralis minor muscle. Subcutaneous tissue and skin are closed with two layers of buried stitches without drainage.

## RESULTS OF TREATMENT

The success rate for pectoralis minor tenotomy (PMT) alone in 52 patients was good in 84%, fair in 8%, and failed in 8% with 1-3 year follow up.[19] (**Sanders 2010**). For patients with both NPMS and NTOS, the results of pectoralis minor tenotomy alone were good in 35%, fair in 19%, failed in 46%.[19] Most of the 65% who were fair or failed underwent thoracic outlet surgery at a later date. In 20 children, the success rate of PMT alone was good to excellent in 75%, fair in 10%, and failed in 15%.[30] (**Sanders 2013**)

# Part II

# Venous Compression: VTOS and VPMS

## CLASSIFICATION

The definition of VTOS is axillosubclavian vein (the main vein of the arm) obstruction with or without clotting. In either case, the symptoms are the same: Arm swelling and arm tightness. The clotting form usually has more intense symptoms than the non-clotting form. Often the symptoms of axillosubclavian vein clotting are preceded by mild symptoms of intermittent obstruction, without clots, so the two conditions should be regarded as progressive stages of the same problem. VTOS or VPMS can also be primary or secondary.

**Secondary venous obstruction** indicates that there is a known cause for the blockage. The most common cause is catheters or wires inserted into the venous system for weeks, months or, in some cases, for years. The catheters are for patients requiring long-term intravenous chemotherapy for infections, cancer, feeding purposes, or for patients with kidney failure who are on renal dialysis. The wires connect implanted pacemakers and defibrillators with the heart, in patients with irregular heart rhythms. The pacemakers are placed under the skin a few inches below the collarbone. Secondary venous obstruction is the more common form of VTOS.

**Primary venous obstruction** is defined as venous obstruction or clotting with no obvious known cause. It is also called Paget-Schrotter Syndrome, [31,32] (**Paget 1875, Schrotter 1884**) effort thrombosis, idiopathic, spontaneous, or traumatic thrombosis. This type is seen more often in teenagers and young adults.

## SYMPTOMS

Symptoms of VTOS or VPMS are swelling and cyanosis (dark red-blue color) of the involved arm. The onset may be sudden, occurring within less than 24 hours; it may also be subtle, occurring over several days. A feeling of tightness is quite common while actual pain may or may not be present. Numbness or tingling is not usually a prominent feature, but is sometimes present when swelling is significant.

**Thrombotic versus non-thrombotic obstruction**: The symptoms of obstruction without clots, are the same as those of obstruction with clots: Swelling and a feeling of tightness in the arm plus cyanosis in the hand and arm. However, in obstruction without clots, the symptoms are intermittent, usually coming with elevation or activity of the arm and receding or even disappearing when the arm is at rest. When clotting occurs, the symptoms are usually more intense and remain constant for days or weeks. They won't disappear quickly unless treated. Failure to treat may result in a permanent, uncomfortable arm presenting with chronic pain, swelling, and dysfunction.

## PHYSICAL EXAMINATION

Swelling of the hand and arm is the primary finding in almost all patients. In some patients, the swelling may be minimal and can only be detected by measuring the circumference of both arms to find an increase in size of as little as 1 cm above and below the elbow.

Color changes in the involved arm are not always present or may be slight. The arm is usually darker in color, often has a blue, dark red, or purplish tinge. The color change is associated with visible, distended veins on the involved arm. Veins are often visible over the shoulder and chest wall of the involved side. This may not be too evident at first glance. To be sure, the veins on the two sides of the chest wall should be compared.

## ETIOLOGY

The body's clotting system is in delicate balance between clot formation and clot dissolving (lysis). Secondary VTOS or VPMS obstruction has several causes that can upset that balance. The most common is the presence of catheters or wires inside the vein. It can also be caused by clotting disorders (coagulopathies), such as Factor 5 deficiency, Protein S or Protein C deficiency, or other types of clotting factor deficiencies or abundance.

Primary VTOS and VPMS were initially regarded as venous obstruction of unknown cause. However, over the past 100 plus years since Paget in 1875[29] and von Schrotter in 1884[30] initially described this condition, much has been learned about the causes of venous obstruction. The anatomy of the subclavian vein as it joins the innominate vein is instructive. The subclavian vein at this point is surrounded by four structures: The first rib below the vein, the subclavius tendon above it, the costoclavicular ligament (CCL) medially (to the inside), and the anterior scalene muscle laterally (to the outside). (**Figure 16**)

## FIGURE16:  RELATIONSHIP OF STRUCTURES SURROUNDING SUBCLAVIAN VEIN

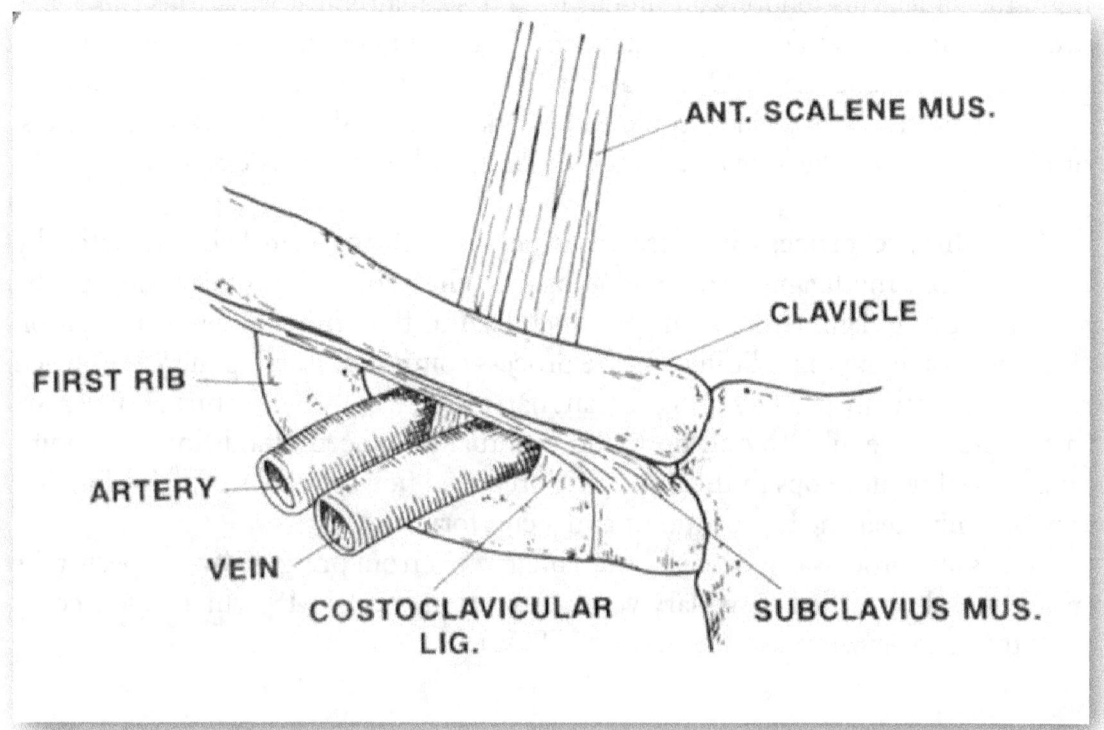

Figure 16: The costoclavicular space. The subclavian vein is bounded by the costoclavicular ligament medially, the anterior scalene muscle laterally, the subclavius muscle tendon superiorly, and the first rib inferiorly.  Reprinted with permission from Sanders RJ, Haug CE: Thoracic outlet syndrome: A common sequela of neck injuries. Philadelphia, Lipppincott, 1991, pg 236

In the early stages of the body's development, if the subclavian vein lies a little too medially, the CCL can indent the vein; if the subclavian vein lies a little too high, the subclavius tendon can indent it. These anatomical variations can act as predisposing causes to develop obstruction if the arm does extensive repetitive activity above shoulder level. Overhead activities that can lead to obstruction include athletes who throw or swim, people who work stocking shelves above their heads, or construction workers or mechanics working with their arms overhead for long periods of time.

**The disease process** in these cases begins with the vein being irritated by pressure from the ligament or tendon against the vein. The inner lining of the vein develops inflammatory changes which lead to thickening and scar formation (fibrosis) inside the vein's lining. As the process continues, scarring increases inside the vein, eventually producing significant narrowing (stenosis). In turn, this results in turbulent (irregular) blood flow, and eventually reduced blood flow to a point where swelling develops in the arm. With reduced flow, platelets and clotting factors organize near the narrow point and a clot forms.

The same process can occur in the axillary vein from pressure by the pectoralis minor muscle resulting in axillary vein obstruction and VPMS, which is less common than subclavian vein obstruction (VTOS).

## DIAGNOSTIC TESTS

**Ultrasound Duplex Scan** is a non-invasive technique that is readily available in most hospitals and in many outpatient medical centers. When it demonstrates total blockage of the axillosubclavian vein it is probably reliable. However, demonstrating flow in the area around the collarbone can be misleading. A large collateral vein (bypassing vein) can be mistaken for the main channel and the diagnosis of subclavian vein thrombosis missed. In such situations, venography (x-ray with dye injected into the vein) will be more dependable.

**Venography**, injecting dye into the basilic vein of the symptomatic arm is the more reliable diagnostic test for axillosubclavian vein obstruction. If injection is through the cephalic vein, a major segment of vein can be bypassed and only the subclavian-innominate vein section seen. **(Figure 17)** In the majority of patients, the main pathology will be in this area and will be detected with a cephalic vein injection. However, when a cephalic vein injection is completely normal while clinically obstruction is suspected, attempts to obtain a basilic vein injection should be made. The use of ultrasound to find a deep-lying vein leading into the basilic system should be attempted.

Venography begins with the arm at the patient's side. If it shows total occlusion, additional injections with the arm elevated are unnecessary. If the resting position reveals normal venous flow, dynamic positioning should follow, repeating the injection with the arm at $90^0$ and again at $180^0$. Particularly in patients with non-thrombotic obstruction, the venogram may be completely normal at rest but demonstrate narrowing or occlusion when the arm is elevated. **(Figure 18A & B)**

Patients who are allergic to injectable iodine can be treated with a steroid preparation prior to the injection. This has helped many patients avoid reactions which they had experienced previously.

Magnetic resonance angiography (MRA) is a second choice. Although MRA can reveal an open or occluded venous system, it does not give the details sometimes needed to plan treatment. However, it can be a good screening technique along with providing information about other areas.

## FIGURE 17: VENOGRAM INJECTING CEPHALIC VEIN AND BYPASSING BRACHIAL AND AXILLARY VEINS

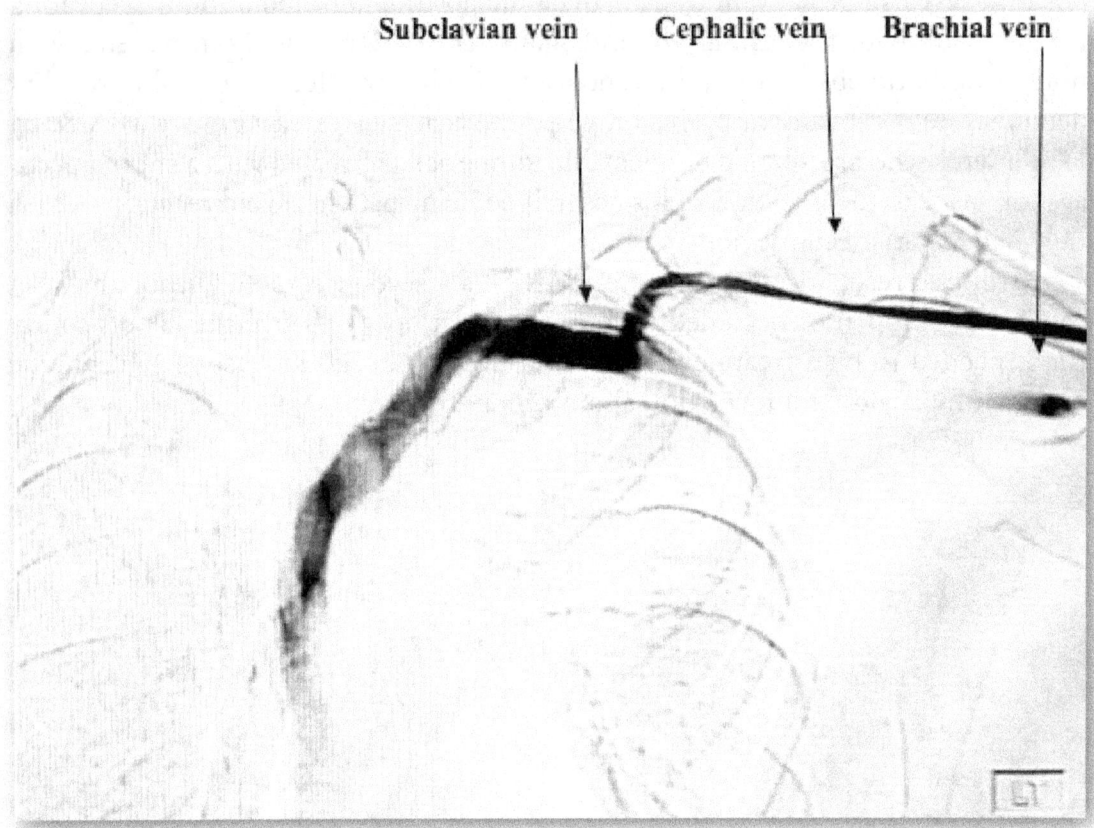

Figure 17: Venogram with injection into the cephalic vein. Note that this bypasses the main brachial and axillary veins, filling only the subclavian vein. (Figure 18 shows these.) To avoid this bypass, the injection into the arm should enter the basilic vein system.

## FIGURE18 A.  VENOGRAM SHOWING OPEN BRACHIAL, AXILLARY, AND SUBCLAVIAN VEINS

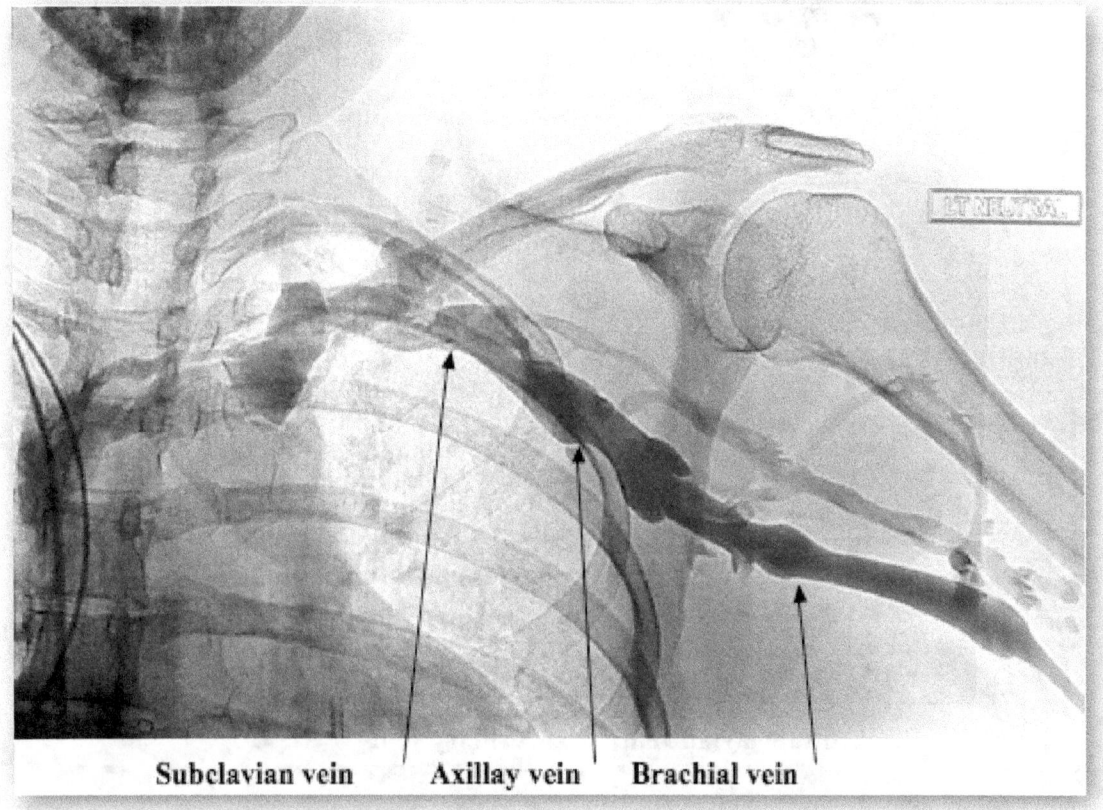

Subclavian vein     Axillay vein     Brachial vein

Figure 18 A:  Venogram with arm at 45 degrees from patient's side, the brachial, axillary and subclavian veins appear normal.

## FIGURE 18 B. ARM ELEVATED, SUBCLAVIAN VEIN OBSTRUCTED

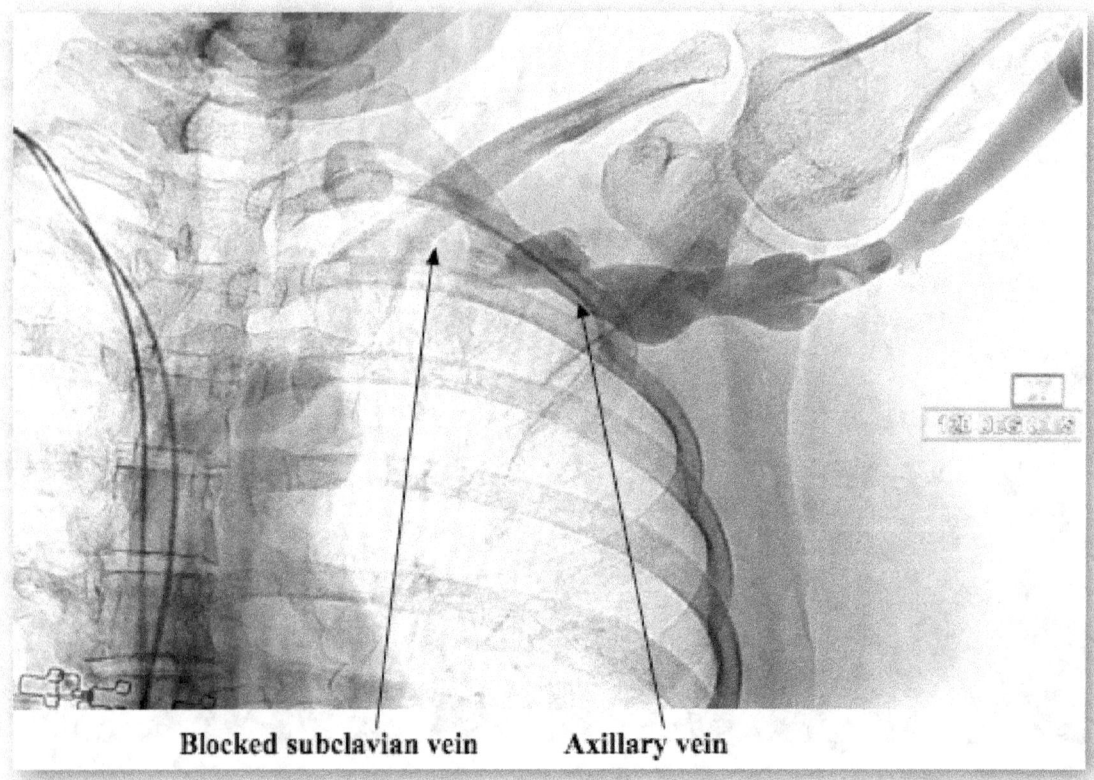

**Blocked subclavian vein**          **Axillary vein**

Figure 18 B:  Same patient as 18A.  With arm elevated to 120 degrees, blood flow is partially obstructed beyond the axillary vein.  The subclavian vein does not fill.  This is non-thrombotic obstruction, there is no clot.

## TREATMENT

Basically, there are two choices of therapy: Anticoagulation or a three step program of thrombolysis, surgery, and possibly balloon angioplasty or vein reconstruction. The choice may be guided by the facilities available to the patient. Rural areas, or areas without medical facilities, may be limited to anticoagulation, if medication is available. Where good medical care is available, the three-step program will lead to faster recovery and less chance of disability.

## VENOUS THORACIC OUTLET SYNDROME (VTOS)

There are 3 steps in treating VTOS.

1. Dissolve the clot by fibrinolysis (dissolving the clot with medication). This is unnecessary if there is no clot. If no clot is present, advance to step two.
2. Treat the extrinsic problem which is the structures outside the vein wall that are compressing the vein. For VTOS these are the first rib, costoclavicular ligament, subclavius tendon, and anterior scalene muscle. For VPMS this is the pectoralis minor muscle.
3. Treat the intrinsic problem if symptoms persist after the extrinsic problem has been resolved. This can be by catheter balloon dilatation (balloon angioplasty) or by surgical venous reconstruction of the residual narrowing or occlusion inside the vein.

### Step 1. Dissolve the clot.

**Acute clotting** of the axillosubclavian vein requires urgent, not emergent, treatment. When a patient presents with a history of recent onset of arm swelling, cyanosis, and tightness or pain in the arm, axillosubclavian vein clotting should be the first diagnosis to consider. The diagnosis can be confirmed with ultrasound duplex scanning. If catheterization and clot dissolving medication can be begun within the next 24 hours, arrangements should be made to do so. Heparin can be started when the patient is initially seen, but it can be delayed 24 hours until the patient is in an appropriate facility.

If facilities for catheter thrombolysis are not readily available, alternative therapy is anticoagulation (blood thinning). Subcutaneous heparin and warfarin are started immediately. This therapy is not as successful as thrombolytic therapy, but it will suffice until thrombolysis is available and can be started within 10 days. Although some patients have seen their clots disappear on just anticoagulation, the success rate is not as good as with early thrombolysis.[33] (**Heron 1999**) If anticoagulation is the only treatment available indefinitely, warfarin therapy should be continued for 3 to 6 months.

Assuming fibrinolysis is available, hospitalization is usually required for a few days. A catheter is inserted into the **basilic** venous system, using ultrasound to find the vein. The catheter is passed up to the axillary vein and a venogram performed. If the catheter enters the cephalic vein instead of the basilic vein, it may bypass some of the clot and give misleading information.

If a clot is demonstrated, the catheter is buried in the clot and thrombolysis begun by continuous drip directly into the clot. Heparin is also started intravenously to prevent extension of clot in the involved arm which can form around and distal (down stream) to the catheter. A venogram is performed at regular intervals to follow the progress of clot dissolution. It may take up to 24 hours to dissolve the clot. Success rate is 62%-84%.[34,35] (**Beygui 1997, Doyle 2007**)

If the clot persists, thrombolytic therapy is stopped after 24-48 hours. When thrombolysis fails to dissolve the clot, breaking up the thrombus with a clot buster can be attempted employing a rotational mechanical thrombectomy device catheter (**Helix**[R]). The use of pharmaco-mechanical thrombectomy may improve patency (opening) and reduce costs. [36,37] (**Lin 2006, Malgor 2012**) One study noted that for clots older than six weeks, only 50 % could be partially opened, none were completely opened. [35] (**Doyle 2007**)

If clot dissolution is unsuccessful, depending on the residual symptoms, the options for further treatment are surgical thrombectomy (removal of clot) with a patch graft or anticoagulation therapy for 3-6 months. (A patch graft is a small piece of material used to close an incision in a blood vessel to avoid narrowing the blood vessel which may happen if the two sides of the open vein are simply sewn to each other.) Venography is helpful in deciding the next step.

It also should be noted that many patients treated with long-term anticoagulation may obtain good relief of symptoms without surgery. This is the result of either the clot dissolving over several weeks to months on long term anticoagulation, and/or the development of good venous collaterals (bypassing veins), which can take several months to develop and mature.

## BALLOON ANGIOPLASTY OR STENTING BEFORE RIB RESECTION

If thrombolysis is successful, the post-thrombolytic venogram is studied. Prior to leaving the catheterization suite, while the catheter is still in place, some physicians will attempt to balloon dilate residual narrowing (angioplasty), as the acute clot has now been dissolved. Angioplasty at this time is occasionally successful. However,

**most of the time, balloon angioplasty fails when it is done before the extrinsic pressure on the vein has been relieved**; the balloon cannot stretch out the tight structures surrounding the vein. In fact, balloon dilatation (enlargement) at this time usually roughens up the vein lining causing inflammation, and may cause the vein to reclot. Our practice is to insert a balloon and inflate it to no more than 6 mm) (this is minimal, capacity is usually over 10mm. This flattens the intima (inner lining of a blood vessel) and any residual clot, but does not attempt to dilate, thus avoiding damage to the vein lining (intima).

Stenting the subclavian vein at this stage also results in a high incidence of failure. Even if stents are employed after first rib resection, stents often fail when placed just below the collarbone. Stents are used only as a last resort and only after the first rib has been removed.

### Step 2. Treat the extrinsic factor

While there is no urgency to perform surgery immediately after successful clot removal, reclotting occurs within four weeks in as many as 30% of patients who initially had successful clot dissolution. Until the external pressure outside the vein wall is relieved, reclotting can occur as nothing has yet been done to remove the underlying cause of the clotting.[38] (**Illig 2010**) The highest success rate is achieved by performing first rib removal and venolysis in the next few days. Until surgery is performed the patient should remain anticoagulated. At the time of surgery, the level of anticoagulation is reduced to lower levels to prevent excessive bleeding during surgery, but not totally stopped (our level is an INR of less than 2.0). Postoperatively, anticoagulation is resumed and continued for 3 months.

Surgical approaches must remove the anterior (front) part of the first rib and cut all ligaments, tendons, and muscles surrounding the subclavian vein. The most popular approach, and the one we prefer, is transaxillary first rib resection through an armpit incision. It also can be done through an incision below the collarbone (infraclavicular approach), although exposure is more difficult going under the collarbone.

**Technique of transaxillary first rib resection**. The operation for VTOS through the armpit is the same as described for NTOS.(**See NTOS-Page 44**) However, after the center of the rib has been removed and the anterior segment removed up to the costal cartilage at the breast bone, additional time is taken to make sure the subclavian vein is totally freed by making sure the costoclavicular ligament and subclavius muscle tendon have been divided and no strands of muscle remain behind the subclavian vein.

## Step 3. Treat the intrinsic factor

Once the first rib has been removed and the subclavian vein freed from extrinsic (outside) pressure, narrowing may still exist inside the subclavian vein lumen (opening). This is determined by postoperative symptoms and venography of the subclavian vein. After decompressive surgery, some patients will have persistent symptoms while others are symptom-free. In the symptom-free patients, a follow up venogram is obtained to make sure there is no significant narrowing. If there is narrowing of less than 50%, nothing further is done except place the patient on therapeutic doses of warfarin for three months and then anticoagulation is stopped. Screening for a clotting disorder may be done if it wasn't done when the patient was first seen, before anticoagulants were administered.

Patients with residual symptoms after surgery, and those who are asymptomatic but have subclavian vein narrowing greater than 50% postoperatively, are treated by balloon angioplasty of the subclavian vein. Now, the vein is much more responsive to dilatation as the extrinsic compressing structures have been removed. Stenting should still be avoided unless absolutely necessary as following stenting, reclotting has been reported as high as 40%.[39] (**Perler 1986**)

## Anticoagulation

Anticoagulation is an alternative to thrombolysis followed by first rib resection. It is also a supplement to the three-step approach. After each step there is usually a raw surface on the vein lining, inside of the subclavian vein. While this will eventually heal with a new, smooth lining (endothelialize), until it does, the vein is at risk to reclot. Therefore, the patient is anticoagulated between steps and after any reconstruction or bypass procedure. (**Figure 19**)

Anticoagulation is begun with heparin or one of its derivatives. Warfarin is also started. Prothrombin times are checked regularly and when the prothombin time reaches an effective, but safe level, the heparin is stopped.

In patients being treated with anticoagulation alone, which for most patients is for 3 to 6 months. However, some studies have shown that maintaining anticoagulation for 12 months improves the success rate.[40] (**Chest 2012**)

FIGURE 19: ALGORITHM OF MANAGEMENT OF VENOUS TOS

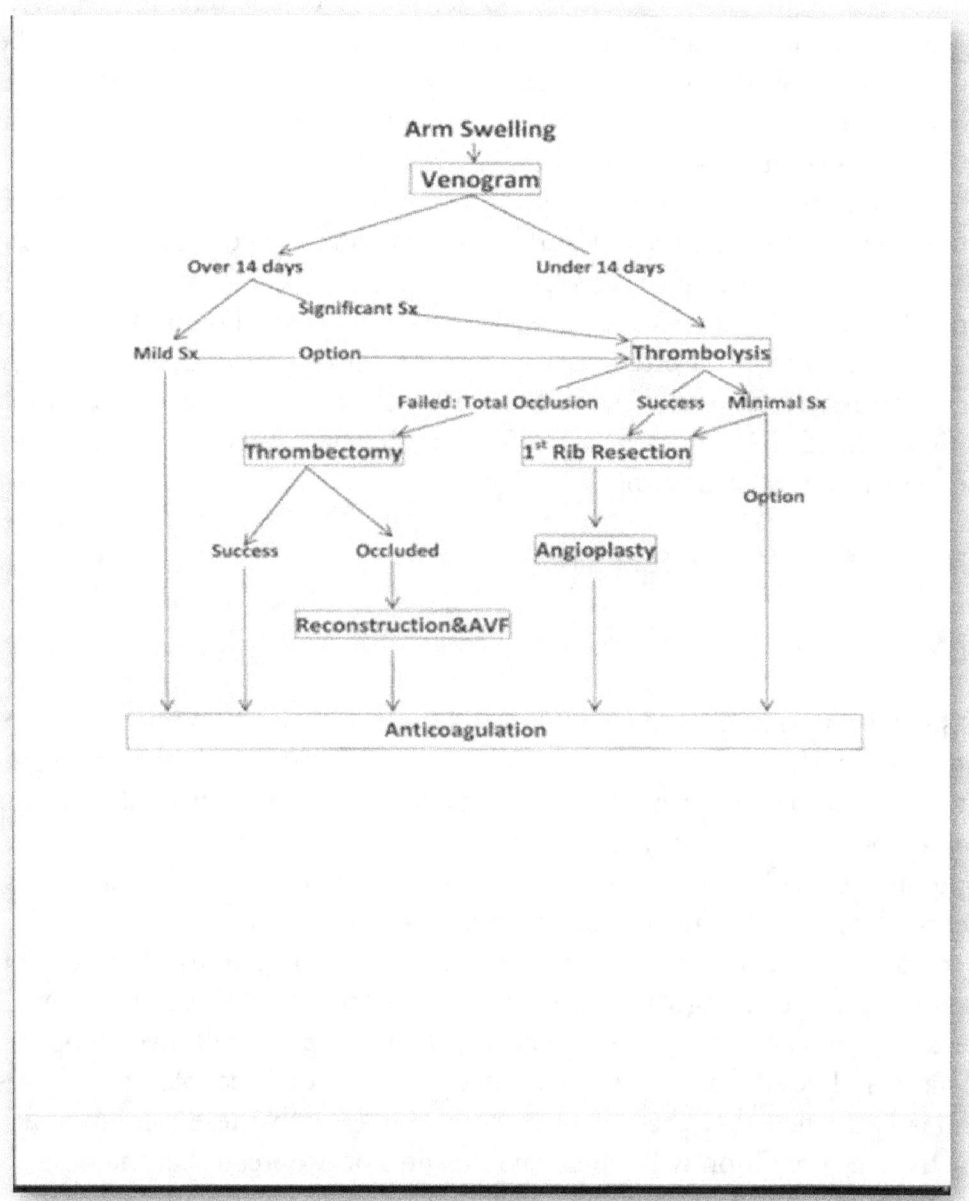

Figure 19: Algorithm of management of venous thoracic outlet syndrome. The length of time after the first swelling is important in the choices of therapy and the results of treatment.

## RESULTS

The success rate for treatment of VTOS depends upon the time interval between the onset of symptoms and the beginning of treatment. Treatment that begins within a few days of the onset of arm swelling has at least a 90% chance of the clot being dissolved and the symptoms gone. [32] Even if treatment is begun within the first 7-14 days of the onset of arm swelling, there is a high success rate.

If the time from the onset of symptoms until treatment begins is longer than 14 days, the success rate is less, but there still are some successes. Lytic therapy is still worth trying if the clot is less than 30 days old, but the greater the delay, the poorer the results. Patients seen after 30 days, or those who failed to open their subclavian veins with lytic therapy, are put on long-term anticoagulation for at least 6 months at therapeutic levels. Studies have shown that the longer the patient is anticoagulated the higher the success rate. However, there is not much further improvement after 3-6 months.

## VENOUS RECONSTRUCTION

### Chronic Venous Obstruction: Postphlebitic and Non-thrombotic (without clot)

Persistent symptoms of arm swelling, tightness, and even paresthesia occur in some patients who have had their acute clotting treated only with anticoagulants. Included in this patient group are those who have undergone first rib removal and venolysis but have reclotted their axillosubclavian vein. In some patients these symptoms exist with venous narrowing but no history of ever having a clot. These patients all fit into the category of chronic venous obstruction.

Treatment depends on the intensity of the symptoms and to what extent these symptoms are interfering with patients' lives. A variety of therapies are available to restore venous blood flow to the arm, but these options all involve operations and successful results are never guaranteed. In general, people whose lives are sedentary may feel that they can live comfortably with these symptoms if they know that the condition will remain stable and not progress. On the other hand, people who are physically active and wish to participate in strenuous work or recreational activities, will often ask if something can be done to improve the use of their arms. Approaches available are: Endovenectomy, bypass grafting, or interposition grafting.

A preoperative venogram is essential to define the area and extent of venous obstruction. In cases where there is only partial venous obstruction, it is sometimes hard to determine exactly where the narrowing is located. In these situations, subtraction techniques to remove the bone from the x-ray images are helpful. (Figures 17 is subtraction technique). The use of real-time video may also demonstrate the point of dye holdup that can be difficult to determine from single exposures. If first rib removal and venolysis have not yet been performed, they should be done either prior to or along with the endovenectomy. This step is not necessary if an axillojugular vein bypass is to be done for total subclavian vein occlusion.

## Subclavian Vein Thrombectomy/Endovenectomy with Vein Patch Closure

The requirements to perform an operation for chronic obstruction of the subclavian vein are a patent axillary vein and internal jugular vein plus significant symptoms interfering with activities of work, sleep, or recreation. Review of the venogram is essential for selecting and planning the best procedure.

The simplest form of venous repair is to open the vein, remove fresh clot, cut out (excise) the scarred, thickened intima (vein lining), and close the vein with a patch so the vein isn't narrowed again by closure of the venous incision. This can be done through an infraclavicular incision. It can also be performed by removing the collarbone, which provides much better exposure, but claviculectomy is rarely done because it can be disabling for active people.

# FIGURE 20: SUBCLAVIAN ENDOVENECTOMY

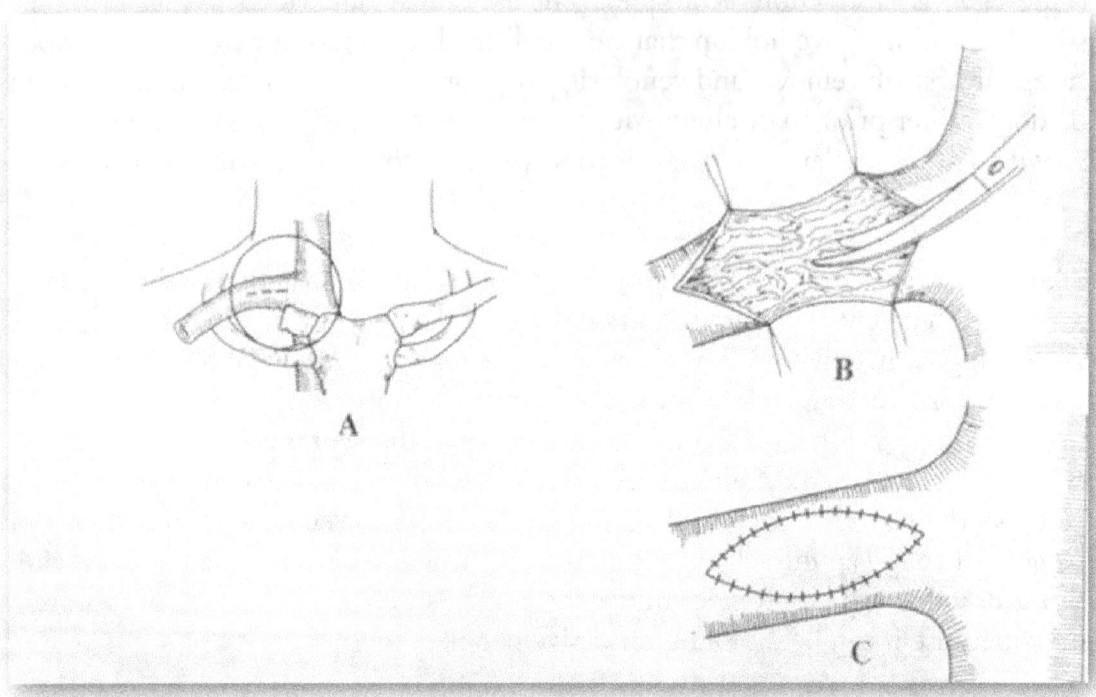

Figure 20: Subclavian vein endovenectomy. A. The skin incision is 2 cm below the collarbone. The pectoralis major muscle is split between its two halves. The subclavian vein is mobilized, occluded with clamps proximally and distally, and an incision is made into the vein. Stitches in the edges of the cut vein hold the vein open to permit removal of the scar tissue. B. Thickened intima is cut out sharply leaving about 1-2 mm of scar to avoid puncturing the vein wall. C. Patch graft closure with autogenous vein or prosthetic material. Reprinted with permission from Sanders RJ, Haug CE: Thoracic outlet syndrome: A common sequela of neck injuries. Philadelphia, Lipppincott, 1991, pg 252

**Technique**: The procedure is performed by exposing the subclavian vein through an 8-10 cm incision about 2 cm below, and parallel to, the collarbone and beginning 3-4 cm from the midline. The venous pathology (disease) usually begins near the costoclavicular ligament close to the subclavian-innominate vein junction. The pectoralis major muscle is split in the direction of its fibers to find the subclavian vein, which may be tucked under the collarbone. The vein is mobilized from the costal cartilage to as far laterally (to the outside) as needed until the soft, uninvolved segment of axillosubclavian vein is identified. The patient is heparinized and plastic vessel loops or vascular clamps used to occlude the involved vein segment. If a fresh clot exists, it is easily flushed out. If a fresh clot exists in the distal vein (down stream), it can be removed with a balloon catheter or thrombectomy forceps. After all fresh clots have been removed, the thickened intima (lining) must be carefully excised (removed) by sharp dissection. Venous intima cannot be treated by the same techniques employed for removing plaque from arteries. No plane of dissection can be developed between intima and adventitia of a vein (the inner lining and the outer layer of the vein wall). The scarred intima must be ecut out sharply, usually with a scissors, taking special care not to cut through the outer vein wall. This usually means a little scar must remain against the wall to keep the wall intact. The vein is closed with a patch of saphenous vein or similar suitable material. (**Figure 20**)

In patients whose disease process extends so far proximally (towards the heart) that control cannot be obtained through the infraclavicular incision, exposure of the more proximal vein can be obtained by splitting the sternum from manubrium to the first interspace, then opening the interspace laterally, far enough to lift the collarbone and costosternal junction. This provides excellent exposure of the innominate-subclavian vein junction with the internal jugular vein.[41] (**Molina 1998**)

The approach described here for chronic venous occlusion is applicable to acute venous thrombosis, particularly when fibrinolysis has failed.

## Claviculectomy

Although removing the collarbone provides the best exposure of the subclavian vein, it is rarely performed because of its cosmetic defect and because it partially destabilizes the shoulder girdle. Twice we have performed claviculectomy (removing collarbone), both times in patients weighing over 300 pounds. Both patients had successful outcomes but some instability of the shoulder girdle. A long term follow up of patients undergoing claviculectomy found objective deficits in mobility and strength, although most of these patients had normal self-perceptions of overall health and upper extremity function.[42] (**Rubright 2013**) (**Figure 21**)

## FIGURE 21: CLAVICULECTOMY

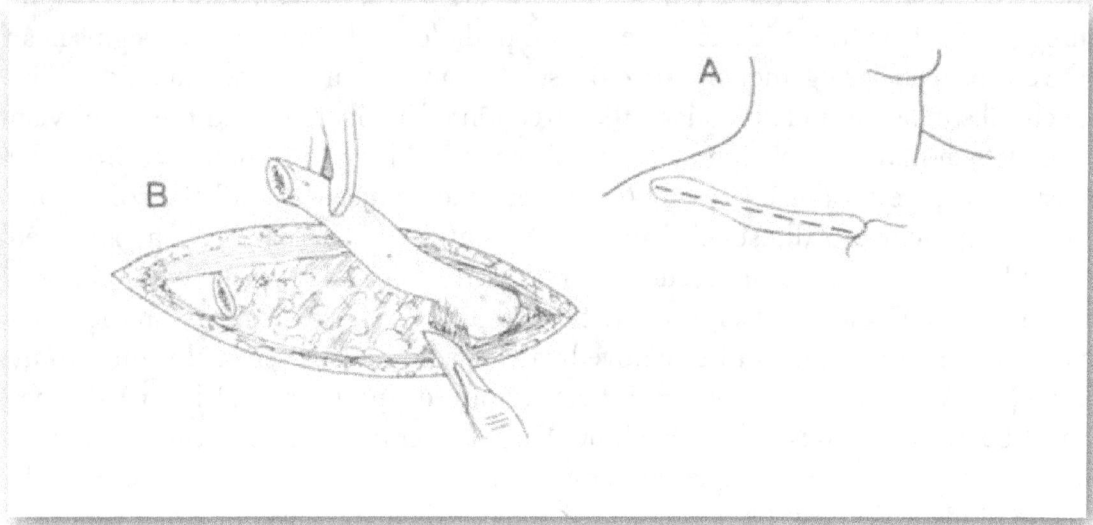

Figure 21: Claviculectomy. A. The incision is made directly over the collarbone. B. The collarbone is dissected circumferentially and divided at least two-thirds of the way towards the acromium process (the end of the collar bone). The medial (inner) two-thirds is elevated and the inner end is disconnected from the joint where the collarbone joins the breast bone (the sternium).

Axillojugular Subclavian Bypass (or axillojugular vein transposition)
The alternative to axillosubclavian vein endovenectomy (**Figure 20**) is to bypass the occluded subclavian vein. The best conduit for this is the internal jugular vein (in the neck) because of its large diameter and convenient location. The indications to perform a bypass are chronic obstruction of the subclavian vein, an open axillary vein into which to sew the internal jugular vein, and significant symptoms interfering with activities of work or recreation. If the axillary vein is also occluded, the bypass is not an option because the internal jugular vein will not stretch much further laterally than the beginning of the axillary vein. In such circumstances, the only alternative is an interposition graft to replace the the section of vein that is cut out..

**Technique**: The incision is about the same as for endovenectomy of the subclavian vein except it is a little more lateral (to the outside) than for subclavian vein endovenectomy because the subclavian vein does not require opening. The venous incision will be in the axillary vein or distal subclavian vein

Once the axillary vein is isolated, the internal jugular vein is mobilized circumferentially (around all sides) through two transverse neck incisions. The internal jugular vein is freed as high as possible, up to the bottom of the skull, where it is suture ligated (tied off). Before dividing it, the anterior surface is marked with a stitch, to prevent twisting when the internal jugular vein is brought down to the axillary vein.

The space below the lower transverse neck incision is dissected down to the collar bone and the internal jugular vein is mobilized all the way to the subclavian-jugular junction near the innominate vein. The subclavius muscle is divided and a portion of it cut out (excised) to create a tunnel through which to pass the divided end of the internal jugular vein to sew it into the axillary vein. (**Figure 22**)

## FIGURE 22. AXILLO-JUGULAR VEIN BYPASS

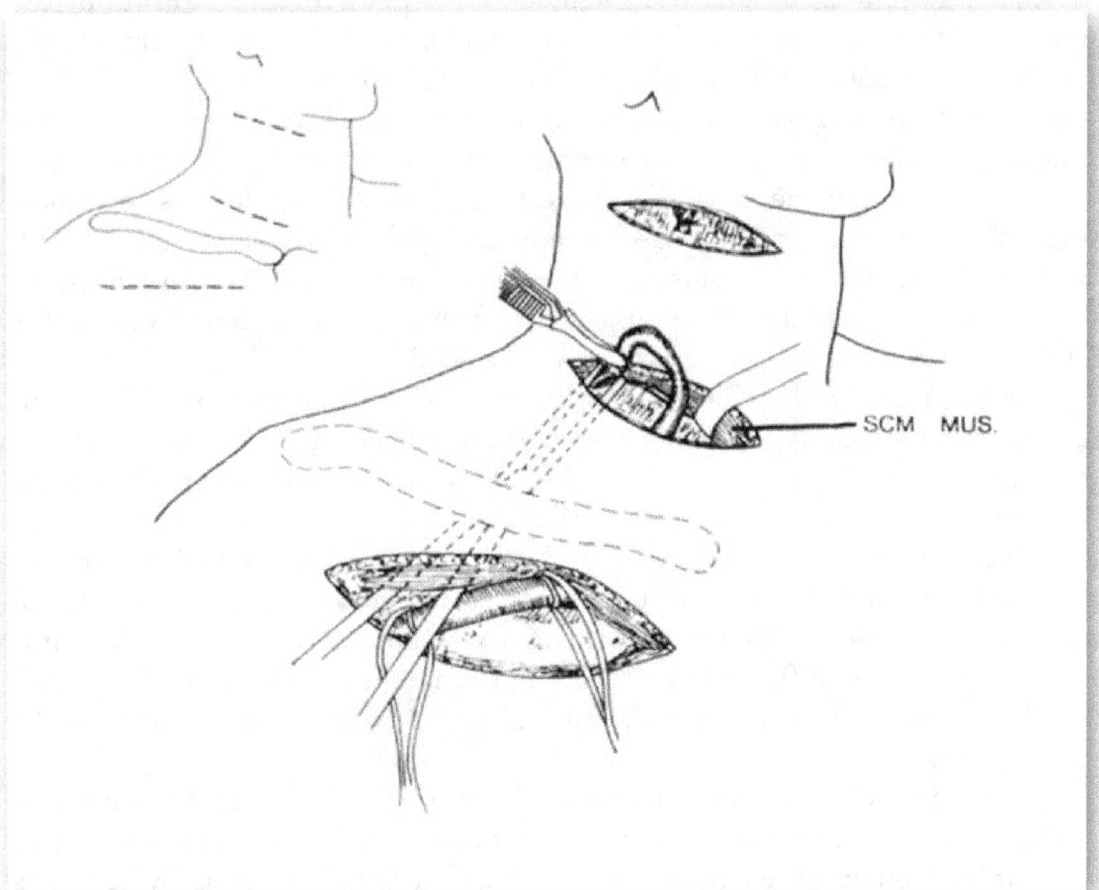

Figure 22: Axillo-jugular vein Bypass . Left:  Placement of the three incisions.  Right: The internal jugular vein has been dissected free, suture-ligated (tied off with a stitch) at the base of the skull, and passed down, below the skin, to the lower neck incision.  The vein is being passed through the tunnel below the collarbone into the lower incision.  The axillosubclavian vein has been freed in preparation for the axillojugular anastomosis  (where two blood vessels are sewn together). Reprinted with permission from Sanders RJ, Haug CE. 1 Subclavian vein obstruction and thoracic outlet syndrome. Ann Vasc Surg 1990;4:397-410.

The internal jugular vein is now brought down in the neck and passes through the tunnel below and behind the collarbone to comfortably reach the axillary vein. Care is taken not to twist the internal jugular vein in its path by observing the marking stich placed in its anterior wall before dividing it. A final check on orientation of the internal jugular vein can be made by passing a small plastic catheter (intra-tracheal catheter) through the open end of the internal jugular vein to make sure it passes smoothly into the innominate vein before the internal jugular vein is sewn in place.

Once this is complete, the patient is heparinized and the (**Figure 22**) subclavian vein is ligated just at the central end (proximal end) of the anastomotic site so blood doesn't collect and clot in the proximal blind stump. The axillary vein is incised (cut open) on its upper surface to receive the internal jugular vein in end-to-side fashion using fine non-absorbable suture. (**Figure 23**)

Alternatively, the anastamosis can be end–to-end. Once completed, the anastamotic site is marked with a metal staple for future x-ray purposes.

# FIGURE 23: COMPLETED SUBCLAVIAN VEIN BYPASSED

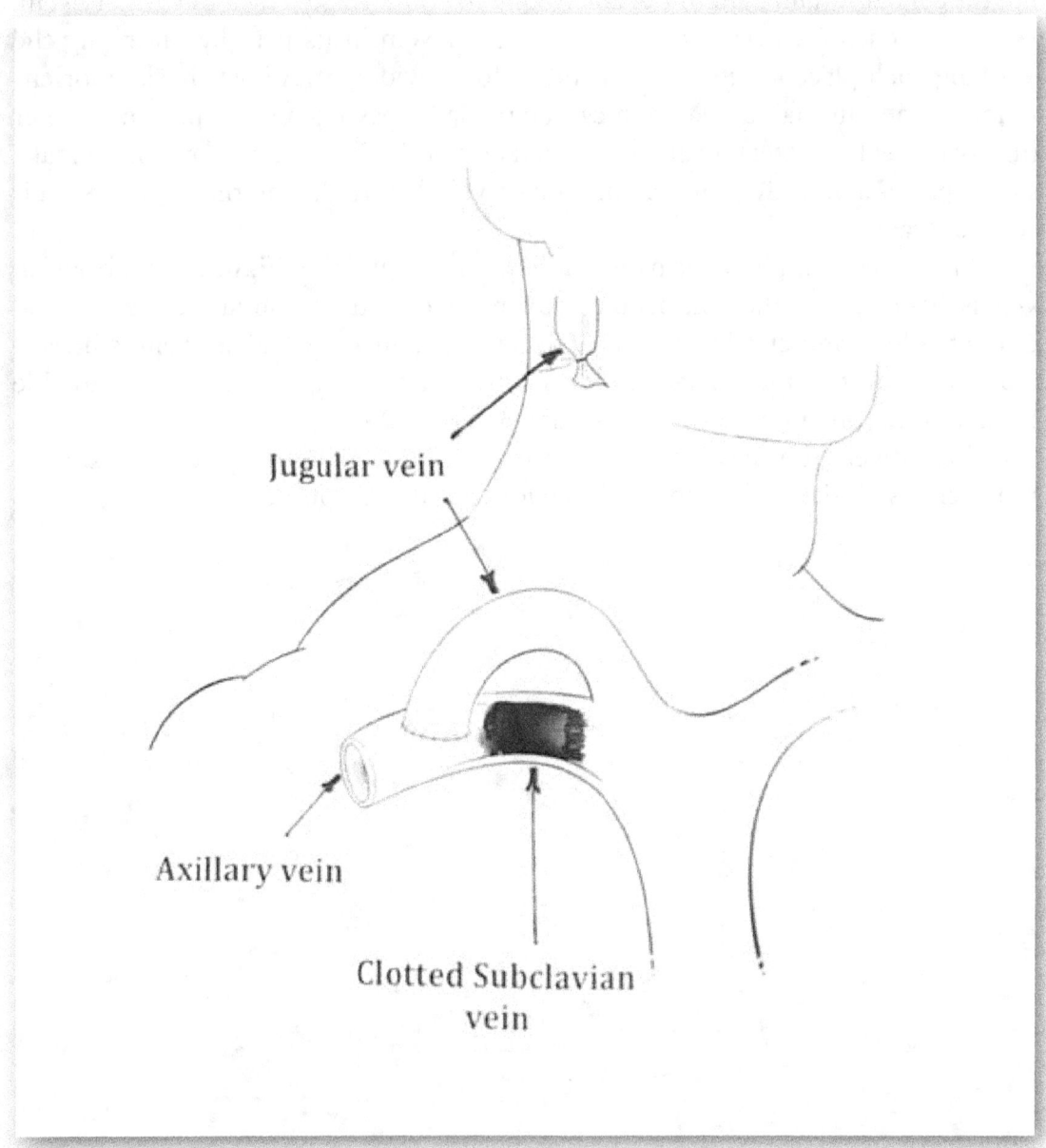

Figure 23: Completed sewing of the jugular vein to the axillary vein and thereby bypassing the subclavian vein occlusion.

**Arteriovenous fistula (AVF)**: Use of an AVF to enhance patency (staying open) after venous repairs was nicely shown by an experiment in dogs and one patient. Venous repairs were demonstrated to have a much higher success rate than controls when an AVF was placed just distal to (beyond) the venous repair. [43] **(Johnson 1969)**

A temporary arteriovenous fistula (AVF) is created distal to the anastamosis (place where two vessels are sewn together) to increase the pressure and flow in the venous system beyond the juguloaxillary anastomosis. Because venous surgery is in a low pressure system, venous repairs or bypass grafts have a greater tendency to clot than do such repairs in the arterial systems which have much higher pressure. By inserting a temporary AVF beyond the site of an endovenectomy or venous bypass, the venous pressure across the raw suture lines is increased. This helps prevent platelets and other clotting elements from collecting at the surgical sites inside the vein. The suture lines and raw surfaces of endovenectomy sites are usually covered with an endothelium (thin lining) within a few weeks, so it is safe to close the fistula after 2-3 months.

For venous repairs in the axillosubclavian vein area, two types of AVF's have been used. One AVF is between axillary artery and axillary vein, just beyond the anastomosis. A stiff, ringed graft of plastic material is used. The graft is looped up to the subcutaneous tissue, just below the skin, so when it is closed, 2-3 months later, it can easily be found and divided. (**Figure 24**) It is unnecessary to remove the pieces of the graft down to their origin. The ends of the plastic graft material have caused no problems after being followed for many years after surgery.

The other type of AVF is a forearm construction, just like the AVF's that are created for renal dialysis. These are easily closed when no longer needed.

FIGURE 24:  VENOGRAM OF COMPLETED
AXILLO-JUGULAR VEIN BYPASS WITH AVF

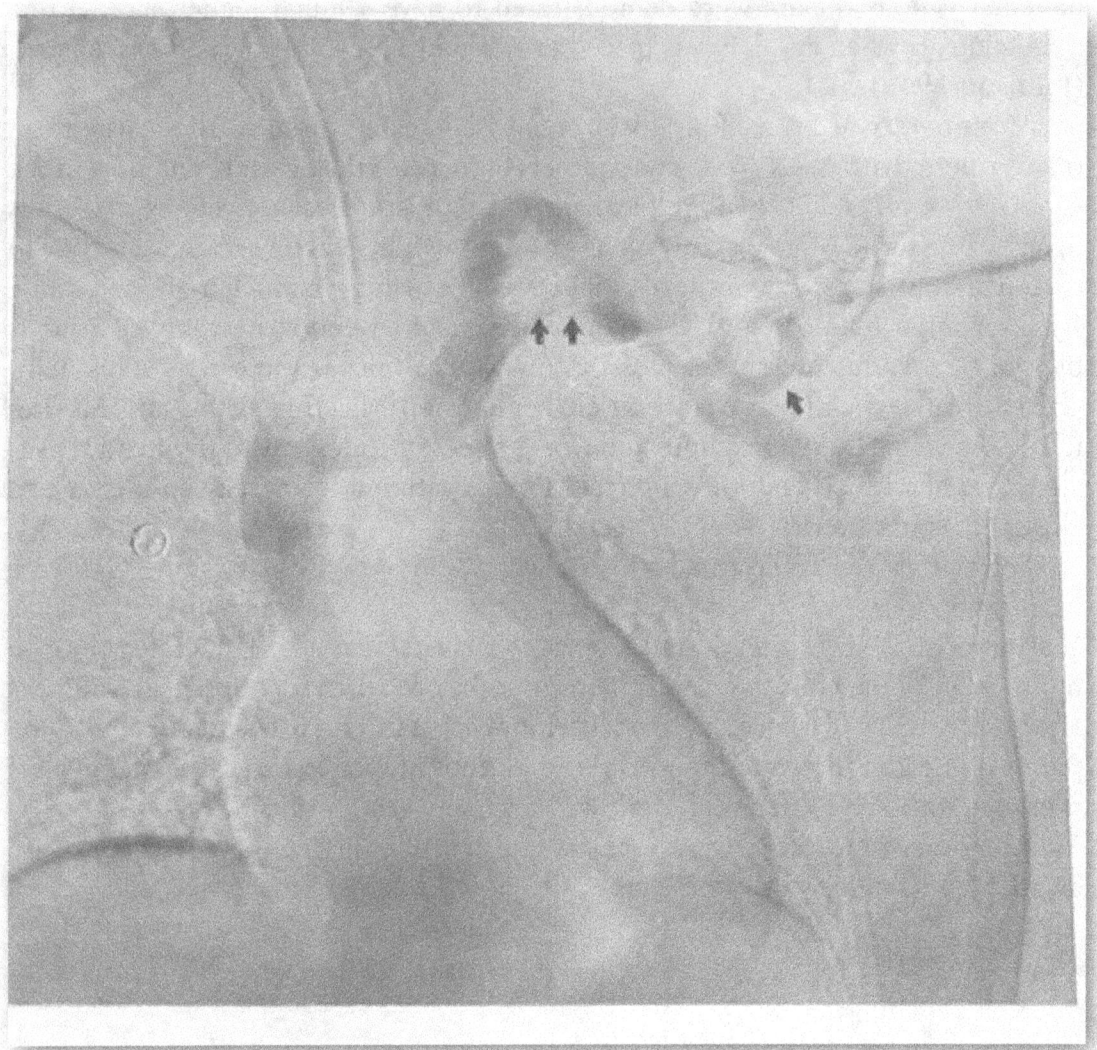

Figure 24:    Venogram of completed axillojugular vein bypass (double arrows) with a
temporary arteriovenous fistula (single arrow).

## THE OPPOSITE SIDE

Patients with unilateral symptoms of subclavian vein compression have a high instance of bilateral subclavian vein compression. In a study of 15 patients with unilateral symptoms of subclavian vein compression, bilateral venograms demonstrated narrowing of the subclavian vein in 80%.[44] (**Kunkel-1989**) As a result, any patient we evaluate for subclavian vein obstruction has bilateral dynamic venography performed. The incidence of symptoms developing in the asymptomatic opposite arm is at least 15%. Patients are presented with the findings on the other side. Some patients will decide that they don't want to go through another clot in their other subclavian vein and will elect a prophylactic (preventitive) first rib resection and venolysis. To date we have not seen another study of the incidence of clotting in the opposite arm. We have not seen any symptoms develop in the patients who underwent prophylactic first rib resection.

# Venous Pectoralis Minor Syndrome (VPMS)

## DEFINITION

It is hard to distinguish the transition from subclavian vein to axillary vein because there is no sharp change in vessel size as there is, for example, between common femoral vein and superficial femoral vein. At the axillosubclavian vein division there is no significant branching to signal a change. The best marker is the pectoralis minor muscle. The axillary vein is defined as that portion of vein lying under the pectoralis minor muscle. Compression of the axillary vein by the pectoralis minor muscle is the definition of VPMS.

## INCIDENCE

VPMS is rare. The first time a series appeared was in 2007 when seven instances of VPMS in six patients were reported.[45] **(Sanders 2007)** Prior to that date there had been only four individual case reports. The only recognized cases have been axillary vein obstruction without thrombosis. Axillary vein clotting alone, without subclavian vein clotting, has not been reported. Of course, clotting of the entire axillosubclavian vein is treated essentially as subclavian vein occlusion. In these cases, the axillary vein involvement is not a separate issue.

## SYMPTOMS

Arm swelling, pain, and cyanosis are the only symptoms of axillary vein obstruction. However, most of the patients seen with VPMS also had additional symptoms of nerve compression, the most common being weakness, numbness, and tingling. This is not surprising as pressure by the pectoralis minor muscle is against the axillary nerves and blood vessels. Because some of the branches of the brachial plexus are very near the axillary vein, it is only natural that nerve symptoms accompany venous ones. Arterial symptoms of arm claudication (pain on exercise) and ischemia are not seen with VPMS as the artery usually lies deep to the vein in the subpectoral space (below the pectoralis minor muscle).

## PHYSICAL EXAMINATION

The only findings on physical examination are mild arm swelling and sometimes distended arm veins and cyanosis. This is not as extensive as the swelling seen with subclavian vein obstruction. All of the findings are subtle and mild.

## ETIOLOGY

There is no clear-cut single cause that has been recognized as the etiology of VPMS. It may be linked to neurogenic PMS where the etiology is often repetitive activities of the upper extremities that require pulling back the shoulder blade, such as weight lifting, throwing, swimming, and similar sports. This causes nerve symptoms more often than venous ones, but the two conditions are often linked together.

## DIAGNOSTIC TESTS

**Venography** is the only diagnostic test that can differentiate subclavian vein from axillary vein compression. Duplex scanning is usually not helpful, as it can't distinguish axillary vein occlusion alone from axillosubclavian vein occlusion.

Venography is helpful in that it can detect various degrees of partial obstruction of the axillary vein, but even this is difficult. We have found the most effective technique is to perform video angiography while the arm is moved through dynamic positions from resting at the side to $180^0$ abduction.

## TREATMENT

Surgery is the only effective treatment for axillary vein obstruction. Pectoralis minor tenotomy (**Page 52**) can be performed through incisions below the collarbone or through the armpit. Our preference is for the transaxillary route. Through this approach it is possible to divide any bands of tight clavipectoral fascia as well as any anomalous bands of muscle, or Langer's arch,[19] which on occasion can compress the axillary vein and branches of the brachial plexus.

# Part III

# Arterial Compression (ATOS and APMS)

## ANATOMY

The subclavian artery exits the thoracic outlet in front of the nerves of the brachial plexus between the scalene muscles in the scalene triangle (**Figure 1B**). It travels over the first rib, beneath the collarbone, and is renamed the axillary artery (**Figure 2**). The axillary artery travels deep to the pectoralis minor muscle where it is surrounded by the nerves of the brachial plexus. It next becomes the brachial artery.

Cervical ribs or anomalous first ribs (**Figure 3**) occur in less than 1% of the population and can compress the subclavian artery and adjacent nerves in the scalene triangle. In the space between collar bone and first rib, the costoclavicular space, a fracture of the collarbone or first rib forming callus (enlargement of new bone at a fracture site) can compress the subclavian artery.

Under the pectoralis minor muscle itself, compression can occur from an over-developed muscle in high performance athletes. The pectoralis minor tendon has been reported to compress and occlude the second portion of the axillary artery [46] (**Finkelstein 1993**). Just distal to the pectoralis minor muscle, the artery can be tethered by the muscle and arterial branches. With extremes of hyperabduction and external rotation, as in overhead pitching, the head of the humerus (upper arm bone) can injure the artery.

The axillary artery has 6 branches, one proximal to (in front of) the pectoralis minor muscle, two deep to the muscle belly, and three beyond the lateral (outer) border of the muscle. The posterior circumflex humoral artery, arising from the distal portion of the axillary artery, and traversing the quadrilateral space, (between teres minor, teres major, long head of the triceps, and humerus) can be compressed along with the axillary nerve. (**Figure 25**)

# FIGURE 25: QUADRALATERAL SPACE

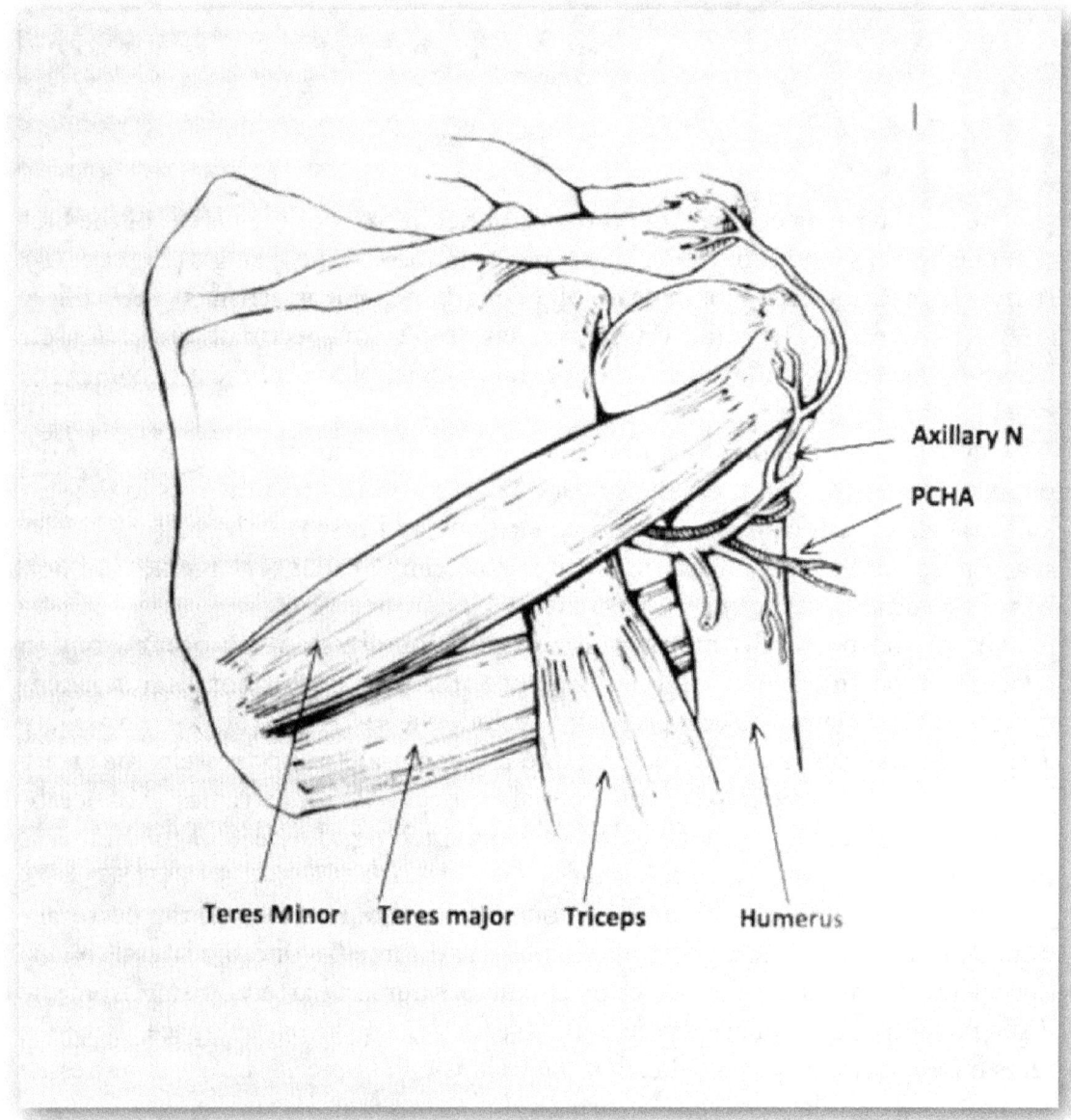

Figure 25: Quadrilateral space bounded by teres major below; teres minor above; long head of the triceps toward the inside; and humerus towards the outside. The posterior circumflex humeral artery (PCHA) and axillary nerve wrapping around the head of the humerus.

## ETIOLOGY

In at least 85% of the patients who develop ATOS the underlying cause is a cervical rib or anomalous first rib.[41] (**Sanders 1991**)  These bony structures exert pressure on the subclavian artery, elevating the artery in the neck, and indenting the artery by pushing against the arterial wall. With each heart beat the artery encounters this unyielding bone.  Arm movement increases arterial wall compression.  Over time, injury to the arterial intima (inner lining) occurs, and fibrosis (scarring) of the arterial wall develops causing stricture or narrowing of the arterial lumen (open space inside a blood vessel).  Like rapids in a river, the velocity (speed) of flow increases through the narrowing, resulting in turbulence and vibrations in the arterial wall.

When this turbulence is enough to cause vibrations and a thrill (or murmur) in the arterial wall, the elastic fibers in the middle layer of the wall of an artery are weakened and the wall becomes more distensible, resulting in enlargement of the vessel diameter and aneurysm formation.[48] (**Roach 1963**) Along the inside wall of the aneurysm, clot forms, which is the source of distal embolization (clots that break off and flow down stream to block smaller arteries in the hand). Clot can develop beyond a narrowing, even without aneurysm formation. This too can embolize distally (downstream).  Intimal injury can cause platelet deposition which results in microemboli (tiny blood clots) producing Raynaud's phenomenon and digital ischemia (lack of blood supply) in the presence of palpable pulses.  A narrowed vessel can totally occlude.  This leads to collateral blood flow (flow in blood vessels going around a blocked blood vessel) and milder symptoms in the arm; it can also lead to retrograde (backward) clots with the possibility of cerebral emboli (blood clots to the brain) causing a stroke. Theoretically, a fibrous band arising from an elongated transverse process of C7 (an excessive extension of a normal piece of bone) could cause compression of the subclavian artery as well.

Another osseous (bony) cause of arterial compression can be callous formation (new bone growth at a fracture site) compressing the artery from fractures of the collarbone or first rib.  Normally, elevating the shoulder narrows the costoclavicular space as the collarbone moves backwards.  Callus from these fractures further narrows this space.

Soft tissue causes (not bone) of arterial occlusion can be seen, particularly in athletes with muscular over-development.  The arteries can be compressed by the nearby muscles or ligaments.   The axillary artery can be squeezed by the pectoralis minor muscle, and the posterior humeral artery can be squeezed in the quadralateral space.  Repeated overhead throwing, common to baseball pitchers and volleyball players, can result in injury to the outer portion of the axillary artery by forward displacement of the head of the humerus against the artery during vigorous throwing. The axillary artery or its circumflex humoral or subscapular branches can also be injured.

## SYMPTOMS

Symptoms of arterial TOS (ATOS) and APMS are those of reduced blood flow in one arm. They may be vague, insidious, and undiagnosed until acute clotting and/or emboli occur, causing severe reduction of blood supply to the arm or hand. The typical symptoms are fatigue and Raynaud's phenomenon with pallor (pale, loss of color) and cyanosis (dark red-blue color) of the hand, cold hypersensitivity of hand and fingers, discoloration of fingertips, and digital ulcers. Other milder symptoms in baseball pitchers are decreased arm endurance, finger ischemia, loss of pitch velocity, arm heaviness, and hand coldness and discoloration. Strokes due to retrograde thrombosis with cerebral emboli (blood clots to the brain) are rare, but have been reported.

## PHYSICAL EXAMINATION

A palpable bony mass, sometimes pulsatile, is often felt just above the collar bone. A murmur may be heard in the same space either with the arm at rest or elevated. The brachial, radial, or ulnar pulses may be absent or diminished at rest, or normal at rest, but absent or diminished with arm elevation.

Blood pressure may be reduced compared to the uninvolved arm. A difference in blood pressure of 20mm or more is considered significant. For accuracy, the blood pressure should be taken by the examiner. Digital changes in the nail beds or finger tips may be seen; the hand may be cooler to touch.

Allen's test, performed by Doppler examination of the radial and ulnar arteries, while the opposite artery is occluded, can reveal occlusion of one of those arteries.

## DIAGNOSTIC TESTS

**Pulse-volume recording**: Waveforms are diminished in the arm and forearm distal to (below) the point of narrowing or obstruction. Digital (finger) photoplethysmography (PPG) reveals digital obstruction rather than vasoconstriction in some or all of the digits.

**Duplex-ultrasound** has the advantage of being low-cost, non-invasive, and can be performed in a standing positions. It can show arterial narrowing, with increased velocity of flow through the narrowing. Other findings are mural thrombus (clot), arterial dilatation (enlargement) or aneurysm, or thrombotic obstruction with collateral formation. Repeating the study with dynamic (elevation) positioning may show abnormalities not present at rest.

Imaging studies:

**Plain x-rays** are the simplest imaging studies. These include cervical spine x-rays with front-to-back, lateral and oblique views, and chest x-rays with back-to-front and lateral views, to reveal bony abnormalities of the neck, ribs, and collarbone. This is the easiest ways to find cervical ribs.

**Magnetic resonance angiography** (MRA) can demonstrate impinging soft tissue structures and arterial irregularity or obstruction. Its accuracy is improved by dynamic positioning in resting and elevated positions. Its advantages are that it does not require ionizing radiation and is the best technique to demonstrate soft tissue structures. It does not require iodinated dye. Disadvantages include cost, the need for the patient to lie still for a prolonged period of time, inability to see bony structures, and the need to perform in lying down position. It cannot be performed in patients with metal implants such as hip or knee prostheses. Rarely a clot can be missed.

**Computerized tomographic angiogram** (CTA) has the advantage of excellent arterial visualization, rapid acquisition of images, and demonstration of bony structures in relation to the artery. Here too, dynamic imaging improves accuracy of diagnosis. The disadvantages of CTA include: exposure to ionizing radiation, requirement of an iodinated contrast agent, failure to demonstrate soft tissues as well as MRI, and the reuirement for performing this in a supine position, whereas the symptoms occur when the patient is upright.

**Digital subtraction arteriography** (DSA) is the injection of contrast material directly into an artery. It has the advantage of demonstrating the entire arterial anatomy from shoulder to fingertip and can be used along with intravascular ultrasound to demonstrate subtle arterial wall irregularities. It can be performed with dynamic positioning, and can be included with therapeutic procedures. Disadvantages include invasiveness of the procedure requiring an arterial puncture, the need for iodinated contrast, and radiation exposure.

## TREATMENT

ATOS is a surgical problem. Acute arterial symptoms are an indication for immediate surgical intervention. Delay in treatment can lead to further complications and a worse result.

Treatment includes 3 steps:

1. Remove the cause
2. Repair or replace the injured artery
3. Restore distal circulation to the arm by removing clots down the arm, dissolving clots with thrombolysis, and/or inserting bypass grafts if necessary.

1. Remove the cause by cutting out the abnormal cervical or anomalous first rib, whenever present. If the cause is a hypertrophied muscle, this is excised.

   With subclavian artery pathology (disease), the supraclavicular approach for rib resection allows for complete examination of the artery and its repair or replacement. In some cases after rib removal, the abnormal segment of artery can be resected (removed) and a tension-free, end-to-end anastamosis can be performed. If the length of artery to be resected is too long for an end-to-end anastamosis, an interpositon or bypass graft can be performed by exposing the axillary artery through a second, infraclavicular incision in the same surgical field.

2. For axillary artery repair, an upper arm incision, extended over the lateral border of the pectoralis major muscle, allows exposure and release of the pectoralis minor muscle and ligation of involved branches of the axillary artery and/or repair of the axillary artery.

3. If arterial blood flow to the distal arm or hand has been compromised by emboli (clots), attempts to restore circulation are undertaken during the same repair procedure. The entire upper extremity is prepared and draped into the operating field. The distal brachial artery and origins of the ulnar and radial arteries are exposed at the antecubital fossa (inside of the elbow). With systemic heparinization, Fogarty balloon embolectomy catheters are passed proximally and distally (up and down the arm) to remove clots, with the goal of restoring normal blood flow. After removing clots, arteriograms are performed immediately, on the operating table, to confirm distal patency (open vessel). If the small vessels have not been opened, clot dissolving (thrombolytic) infusion is performed by slow injection into the open vessels which will carry it down to the blocked vessels. This procedure may require 30-60 minutes. In rare cases, a distal bypass graft, from the upper arm to the wrist, may be required to save the hand. After surgery, anticoagulation and antiplatelet therapy may be required. (**Figure 26**)

# FIGURE 26: ALGORITHM OF SEQUENCE
# OF EVENTS IN ARTERIAL TOS

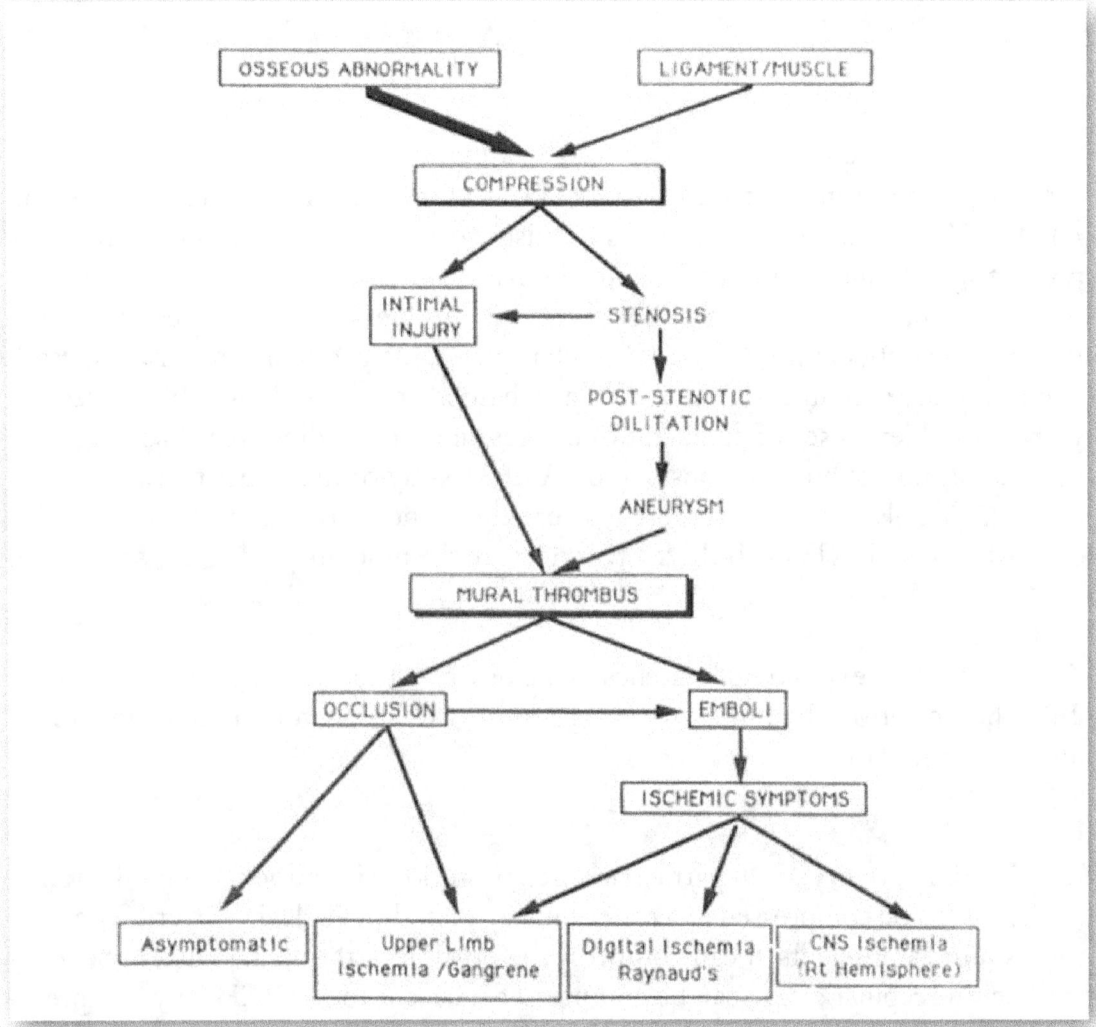

Figure 26: Algorithm of sequence of events in arterial TOS. Most cases are associated with a cervical or anomalous first rib. Intimal injury is the primary pathology.

# Arterial pectoralis minor syndrome--APMS

## INTRODUCTION

Arterial pectoralis minor syndrome (APMS) is a rare condition, seen less often than ATOS. APMS initially is hard to distinguish from ATOS because both conditions present with reduced blood supply to the hand and arm. However, it is very important to determine, as early as possible, if the problem is above the collarbone in the thoracic outlet area or below the collarbone in the pectoralis minor area. Both conditions are seen in athletes, particularly baseball pitchers. If an athlete presents with the sudden onset of pain, color changes, and no swelling in a throwing arm, both conditions should be considered. A plain x-ray of the upper chest and neck can immediately determine if there is a cervical or anomalous first rib. If so consider the diagnosis is ATOS. If the x-ray is normal, the more likely diagnosis is APMS.

## ANATOMY

**The axillary artery** and its branches, were described earlier (**Page 87** and **Figure 25)** The posterior circumflex humeral artery (PCHA) is the branch most often involved in APMS.

## ETIOLOGY AND PATHOPHYSIOLOGY

**The axillary artery**, and particularly its posterior circumflex humeral branch (PCHA), can be compressed in a different way than the subclavian artery. The pectoralis minor muscle itself can compress the portion of the axillary artery beneath it. The subscapular artery can be compressed adjacent to the PCHA by compressing it in the quadralateral space. The head of the humerus can compress the lateral portion of the axillary artery during vigorous throwing. The axillary artery or its circumflex humeral or subscapular branches can also be injured by blunt trauma.

Because the PCHA winds around the humeral head, it can be stretched with forceful overhead motions of the arm. This produces traction at the junction of the PCHA with the axillary artery thereby weakening the wall at this spot. This leads to intimal lesions, aneurysm formation, and subsequent clotting. As overhead action continues, the clot is compressed and portions can enter the axillary artery and be washed downstream as emboli.

## SYMPTOMS

Symptoms of APMS are similar to those of ATOS, but they tend to be more mild and subtle. Some pitchers note a decrease in speed or loss of control while pitching. Coolness in the fingers of the pitching hand and loss of endurance during competition or practice are early signs of axillary artery narrowing resulting in diminished blood flow to the extremity. Arm claudication (pain on exercise), fatigue, and eventually pain, numbness, tingling, and digital ulcerations are evidence of progression. Neurological symptoms of pain and paresthesia may accompany arterial symptoms because the axillary nerve can be compressed in the quadralateral space along with the PCHA.

## PHYSICAL EXAMINATION

The specific findings on physical examination with axillary artery involvement are tenderness just below the collarbone over the pectoralis minor muscle and/or tenderness over the quadralateral space, located just behind the armpit. Radial and/or ulnar pulses may be diminished or absent; blood pressure may be diminished and coolness and color changes may be detected when compared to the good arm and hand.

## DIAGNOSTIC TESTS

The imaging tests for APMS are the same as for ATOS and are described above (**Page 91**). It should be emphasized that detailed views of the axillary artery and each of its branches should be visualized to insure an accurate diagnosis. Although digital subtraction angiography (DSA) is the technique most often employed, in some instances, magnetic resonance angiography (MRA) or computerized tomography angiography (CTA) may provide additional information.

## TREATMENT

Treatment of APMS is less complicated than that for ATOS. In APMS an osseous (bony) cause is not involved; the only pathology is in or around the axillary artery. Angiography that details the specific area to be treated is essential.

    **Thrombolysis,** (dissolving clot) either before or during operative repair, can eliminate clots in the digital vessels. In the operating room, the entire upper extremity should be included in the operative field for possible angiography and thrombolysis via the antecubital space (elbow area).

    **Axillary artery repair** is performed through an upper arm incision, extended over the outerl border of the pectoralis major muscle. This allows exposure and release of the pectoralis minor muscle and ligation of involved branches and/or repair of the axillary artery.

When the pathology is clotting of the posterior circumflex humeral artery, that artery should be divided at or near its axillary artery origin. If the origin encroaches on the axillary artery, as aneurysms can do, repair of the artery with a vein patch will prevent narrowing at this spot in the artery. If the axillary artery is occluded or narrowed over a significant distance, an interposition replacement graft may be required.

**Interposition grafts** in the axillary artery require special attention to insure that the repaired artery will not be reinjured by over-stretching when overhead activity is resumed. In the operating room, the length of the graft should be carefully measured with the arm fully extended. The graft material should be autogenous (the patient's own) vein if at all possible, and the graft should have widely beveled end-to-end anastomoses.[49,50] (**Atema 2012, Duwaryi 2011**) Completion arteriography should be performed immediately after completing the anastomoses.

## RESULTS OF TREATMENT

In a review of 29 published cases of APMS, seven required interposition grafts, eleven were treated with lateral repairs and patch grafts, five were treated with simple ligations of the posterior circumflex humeral artery, five with pectoralis minor tenotomy, and one treated with antiplatelet drugs.[46,49-54] Two patients were operated upon a second time for additional decompression. Twenty-seven of the 29 patients returned to their previous work or competitive sports. The other two were symptom free but retired from their previous activity. There were no amputations and no disability.[55] (Sanders2015)

# References

1. Upton ARM, McComas AJ: The double crush in nerve-entrapment syndromes. Lancet 1973; 2:359-362.
2. Illig KA, Thompson RS, Freischlag JA, Donahue DM, Jordan SE, Edgelow PI, Eds. Thoracic Outlet Syndrome. Springer. London, New York, 2013, pge XIV.
3. Haven H: Neurocirculatory scalenus anticus syndrome in the presence of developmental defects of the first rib. Yale J Bio 1939; 11:443-448.
4. Elvey, RL. The investigation of arm pain. In :Grieve GP, ed. Modern manual therapy of the vertebral column. Edinburgh: Churchill Livingstone, 1986: 530-535.
5. Adson AW, Coffey JR: Cervical rib: a method of anterior approach for relief of symptoms by division of the scalenus anticus. Ann Surg 1927; 85: 839-857.
6. Gergoudis R, Barnes R W: Thoracic outlet arterial compression: prevalence in normal persons. Angiology 1980; 31:538-541.
7. Warrens A, Heaton JM: Thoracic outlet compression syndrome: the lack of reliability of its clinical assessment. Ann R Coll Surg Engl 1987; 69:203-204.
8. Colon E, Westdrop R: Vascular compression in the thoracic outlet: age dependent normative values in noninvasive testing. J Cardiovasc Surg 1988; 29:166-171.
9. Plewa MC, Delinger M: The false-positive rate of thoracic outlet syndrome shoulder maneuvers in healthy subjects. Acad Emerg Med 1998;5:337-342.
10. Nord KM, Kapoor P, Fisher J, Thomas G, Sundaram A, Scott K, Kothari MJ. False positive rate of thoracic outlet syndrome diagnostic maneuvers. Electromyogr Clin Neurophysiol 2008;48:67-74.

11. Nishida T, Price SJ, Minieka MM. Medial antebrachial cutaneous nerve conduction in true neurogenic thoracic outlet syndrome. Electromyogr Clin Neurophysiol 1993; 33:255-258.

12. Kothari MJ, Macintosh K, Heistand M, Logigian EL. Medial antebrachial cutaneous sensory studies in the evaluation of neurogenic thoracic outlet syndrome. Muscle Nerve 1998;21:647-649

13. Seror P. Medial antebrachial cutaneous nerve conduction study, a new tool to demonstrate mild lower brachial plexus lesions. A report of 16 cases. Clin Neurophysiol 2004;115:2316-2322.

14. Machanic BI, Sanders RJ. Medial antebrachial cutaneous nerve measurements to diagnose neurogenic thoracic outlet syndrome. Ann Vasc Surg 2008; 22:248-254.

15. Boulanger X, Ledoux JB, Brun AL, Beigellman C. Imaging of the non-traumatic brachial plexus. Diagn Interv Imaging 2013;94:945-956

16. Filler A. Magnetic resonance neurography and diffusion tensor imaging: origins, history, and clinical impact of the first 50,000 cases with an assessment of efficacy and utility in a prospective 5000-patient study group. Neurosurgery. 2009 Oct;65(4 Suppl):A29-43.

17. Edgelow PI. Physical therapy for NTOS. In Illig et al Eds, Thoracic outlet syndrome. Springer-Verlog London, 2013, Pgs 167-173.

18. Buchanan PA1, Ulrich BD. The Feldenkrais Method: a dynamic approach to changing motor behavior. Res Q Exerc Sport. 2001;72:315-323.

19. Sanders RJ, Rao NM. The forgotten pectoralis minor syndrome: 100 operations for pectoralis minor syndrome alone or accompanied by neurogenic thoracic outlet syndrome. Ann Vasc Surg 2010 24:701-708.

20. Magee C1, Jones C, McIntosh S, Harkin DW. Upper limb deep vein thrombosis due to Langer's axillary arch. J Vasc Surg. 2012;55:234-236.

21. Robicsek F1, Eastman D. "Above-under" exposure of the first rib: a modified approach for the treatment of thoracic outlet syndrome. Ann Vasc Surg. 1997;11:304-306

22. Thompson RW1, Schneider PA, Nelken NA, Skioldebrand CG, Stoney RJ. Circumferential venolysis and paraclavicular thoracic outlet decompression for "effort thrombosis" of the subclavian vein. J Vasc Surg. 1992;16:723-32.

23. Sanders RJ, Pearce WH: The treatment of thoracic outlet syndrome: a comparison of different operations. J Vasc Surg 1989; 10:626-634.

24. Sanders RJ, Roos DB: The surgical anatomy of the scalene triangle. Contemp Surg 1989; 35:11-6.

25. Sanders, RJ, Annest SJ. Technique of supraclavicular decompression for neurogenic thoracic outlet syndrome. J Vasc Surg 2015;61:821-825.
26. Ambrad-Chalela E, Thomas GI, Johansen KH. Recurrent neurogenic thoracic outlet syndrome. Am J Surg 2004; 187:505-510.
27. Sanders RJ. Recurrent neurogenic thoracic outlet syndrome stressing the importance of pectoralis minor syndrome. Vasc Endovascular Surg. 2011;45:33-38
28. Annest SJ, Sanders RJ. Assessment and treatment of recurrent NTOS. In Illig et al Eds, Thoracic outlet syndrome. Springer-Verlog London, 2013, Pgs 281-289
29. Sanders RJ, Hammond SL. Diagnosis of thoracic outlet syndrome. J Vasc Surg 2007; 46: 601-604.
30. Sanders RJ, Annest SJ, Goldson E. Neurogenic thoracic outlet and pectoralis minor syndromes in children. Vasc Endovascular Surg. 2013;47:335-341.
31. Paget J: Clinical lectures and essays. London, 1975.
32. von Schrotter L: Handbuch der allgemeinen pathologie und therapie (Nothnagel). Berlin., A. Hirschwald, 1884. pg 533. Cited by Sampson JJ: Am Heart J 1943; 25:313.
33. Heron E, Lozinguez O, laurian C, Fiessinger JN. Long term sequelae of spontaneous axillary subclavian vein thrombosis. Ann Int Med 1999;131:510-513.
34. Beygui RE, OlcottC 4th, Dalman RI. Subclavian Vein thrombosis: Outcome based on etiology and modality of treatment. Ann vasc Surg 1997;11:247-255.
35. Doyle A, Wolford HY, Davies MT, Adams JT, Singh MJ, Saad WE, et al. Management of effort thrombosis of the subclavian vein: Today's treatment. Ann Vasc Surg 2007;21:723-729.
36. Lin PH, Zho W, Dardik A, Mussa F, Kougias P, Hedayati N, Naoum JJ, El Sayed H, Peden EK, huynh TT. Catheter directed thrombolysis versus pharmacomechanical thrombectomy for treatment of symptomatic lower extremity deep venous thrombosis. Am J Surg 2006; 192:782-788.
37. Malgor RD, Gasparis. Pharmaco-mechanical thrombectomy for early thrombus removal. Phlebology 2012; 27:155-162.
38. Illig KA, Doyle AJ. A comprehensive review of Paget-Schroetter symdrome. J Vasc Surg 2010;51:1538-1547.
39. Perler BA, Mitchell SE. Percutaneous transluminal angioplasty and transaxillary first rib resection. A multidisciplinary approach to the thoracic outlet syndrome. Am Surg. 1986;52:485-488.

40. Antithrombotic Therapy and Prevention of Thrombosis, 9th ed: American College of Chest Physicians Evidence-Based Clinical Practice Guidelines. Chest 2012; supplement.

41. Molina JE: A new surgical approach to the innominate and subclavian vein. J Vasc Surg 1998;27:576-581.

42. Rubright J, Kelleher P, Beardsley C, Paller D, Shackford S, Beynnon, Shafritz A. Long-term clinical outcomes, motion, strength, and function after total claviculectomy. J Shoulder Elbow Surg. 2014;23:236-244.

43. Johnson V, Eiseman B: Evaluation of arteriovenous shunt to maintain patency of venous autograft. Am J Surg 1969; 118:915-920.

44. Kunkel JM, Machleder HI: Treatment of Paget-Schroetter syndrome: A staged, multidisciplinary approach. Arch Surg 1989; 124:1153-1158.

45. Sanders RJ, Rao NM. Pectoralis minor obstruction of the axillary vein: Report of six patients. J Vasc Surg 2007; 45:1206-1211.

46. Finkelstein JA, Johnston KW. Thrombosis of the axillary artery secondary to compression by the pectoralis minor muscle. Ann Vasc Surg. 1993;7:287-290.

47. Sanders RJ, Haug CE: Thoracic outlet syndrome: A common sequela of neck injuries. Philadelphia, Lipppincott, 1991, pg 226

48. Roach MR: Changes in arterial distensibility as a cause of poststenotic dilatation. Am J Cardiol 1963;12:802-815.

49. Atema JJ, Unlu C, Reekers JA, Idu MM. Posterior circumflex humeral artery (PCHA) injury with distal embolizaion in professional volleyball players: Discussion of three cases. Eur J Vasc endovascular Surg 2012;44:195-198.

50. Duwayri YM, Emery VB, Driskill MR, Earley JA, Wright rW, Paletta GAJr, Thompson RS. Position compression of the axillary artery causing upper extremity thrombosis and embolism in the elite overhead throwing athlete. J Vasc Surg 2011;53:1329-1340.

51. Arko, FR, Harris EJ, Zarins CK, Olcott, CIV. Vascular complication in high-performance athletes. J Vasc Surg 2001

52. Schneider K, Kasparyan NG, Altchek DW, Fantini GA, Weiland AJ. An aneurysm involving the axillary artery and its branch vessels in a major league baseball pitcher. Am J Sports Med 1999;27:370-375.

53. Durhan JR, Yao JST, Pearce WH, Nuber GM, McCarthy WJ. Arterial injuries in the thoracic outlet syndrome. J Vasc Surg 1995;21:57-70

54. McCarthyWJ, Yao JST, Schafer MF, Nuber G, Flinn WR, Blackburn D, Suker JR. Upper extremity arterial injury in athletes. J Vasc Surg 1989;9:317-327.

55. Sanders RJ, Annest SJ. Thoracic outlet and pectoralis minor syndromes. Semin Vasc Surg; 2015: June issue. In Press

# Glossary of medical terms and abreviations

**Anomalous first rib**:  abnormal first rib

**Anastamose**:  Sewing together two blood vessels

**Anastamosis**:  The point where two blood vessels are sewn together

**Arteriogram**: X-ray with injection of dye to view circulation in veins.

**Asymptomatic**:  No symptoms

**Axilla:**  Armpit

**Brachial plexus**:  The nerves supplying the arm and hand and located just above and just below the collar bone.

**Callus:**  New bone forming at a fracture site that surrounds the fractured bones

**cm**:  abbreviation for centimeter (about ½ an inch)

**Clavicle**:  Collabone

**Clinical findings**:  Observations based on history and physical examination only, not including any tests.

**Claudication**:  pain in an arm or leg with activity that goes away with rest.

**CNS**:  Central Nervous system (The brain and s[inal cord)

**Collateral**:  Blood vessels that develop to replace circulation around a blocked blood vessel.

**Compression**: Squeezing or applying pressure

**Cyanosis**:  Dark red-blue color

**Decompression**: Relieving pressure by removing scar tissue from a from a blood vessel or nerve

**Dissect:** To cut apart or free up a structure

**Distal**: Away from the center of the body

**EAST**: Elevated arm stress test. This is the "stick-em-up" position (arms above head)

**Emboli**: Blood clots that break off of a larger clot and are carried down stream to block smaller blood vessels.

**Fibrinolysis:** Dissolving the fibrin in the clot. (Fibrin is a main component of a clot)

**Hyperextension**: stretching backwards as in a whiplash injury

**Intima**: Inside lining of any blood vessel

**Ischemia**: Lack of blood supply

**Lysis:** To dissolve a blood clot or remove scar tissue

**mm**: abbreviation for millimeter (between 1/16th and 1/32nd of an inch)

**MRI**: Magnetic Resonance Imaging (A diagnostic test using magnets)

**Mural**: Wall

**Neurologic**: Referring to nerves

**Objective findings**: Measurable test results that don't depend upon the patient's feelings or response.

**Obstruction**: Blocking as blocking blood flow

**Occlusion**: Blockage

**Osseous**: Bony

**Pathology**: Abnormality, disease, or disease process

**Pathophysiology:** describes how symptoms develop from a disease process

**Pectoralis Minor Syndrome**: Symptoms of numbness, tingling and pain in the arm and hand due to pressure against the nerves and/or blood vessels to the arm by the pectoralis minor muscle.

**PMM**: Pectoralis minor muscle

**Pneumothorax:** Air inside the chest collapsing part or all, of the lung.

**Predisposition:** Usually an anatomical variation making someone more likely to develop a specific disease with only mild provocation.

**Provocative maneuvers**: Movements on physical examination that bring out (or provoke) symptoms that are absent when the patient is at rest.

**Proximal**: Closer to the center of the body

**Raynaud's phenomenon**: Coldness and color changes in a hand or foot due to increased sympathetic nerve stimulation. The precise cause is unknown.

**Stenosis**: Narrowing in a blood vessel

**Subclavian Vein and subclavian artery**: The large artery and vein supplying the entire arm.

**Subjective findings**: Results expressed by the patient's feelings in response to a test

**Symptoms**: Complaints

**Trauma**: injury by some type of accident

**Thrombus**: Blood clot

**Thrombolysis**:  Dissolving thrombus or clot with medication or mechanical devices

**Ultrasound Duplex Scan.**  A non-invasive diagnostic tool to visualize blood vessels under the skin.

**ULTT**:  Upper limb tension test—a reliable test for neurogenic TOS and PMS.

**Vascular**:  Referring to blood circulation; a blood vessel, either artery or vein

**Venogram**:  X-ray with injection of dye to view circulation in veins.

**Venolysis**:  Removing all tight structures surrounding a vein.  Around the subclavian vein these are: costoclavicular ligament, subclavius tendon, anterior scalene muscle, and fisrt rib.

www.ingramcontent.com/pod-product-compliance
Lightning Source LLC
Chambersburg PA
CBHW080818180526
45168CB00006B/2493